Stress Management

How to Start Thinking Positively and Overcome Burnout Syndrome

(Easy Ways to Manage Your Daily Stress to Keep You Focused on What Matters to You)

Ralph Souza

Published By **Darby Connor**

Ralph Souza

All Rights Reserved

Stress Management: How to Start Thinking Positively and Overcome Burnout Syndrome (Easy Ways to Manage Your Daily Stress to Keep You Focused on What Matters to You)

ISBN 978-1-7774976-6-8

No part of this guidebook shall be reproduced in any form without permission in writing from the publisher except in the case of brief quotations embodied in critical articles or reviews.

Legal & Disclaimer

The information contained in this book is not designed to replace or take the place of any form of medicine or professional medical advice. The information in this book has been provided for educational & entertainment purposes only.

The information contained in this book has been compiled from sources deemed reliable, and it is accurate to the best of the Author's knowledge; however, the Author cannot guarantee its accuracy and validity and cannot be held liable for any errors or omissions. Changes are periodically made to this book. You must consult your doctor or get professional medical advice before using any of the suggested remedies, techniques, or information in this book.

Upon using the information contained in this book, you agree to hold harmless the Author from and against any damages, costs, and expenses, including any legal fees potentially resulting from the application of any of the information provided by this guide. This disclaimer applies to any damages or injury caused by the use and application, whether directly or indirectly, of any advice or information presented, whether for breach of contract, tort, negligence, personal injury, criminal intent, or under any other cause of action.

You agree to accept all risks of using the information presented inside this book. You need to consult a professional medical practitioner in order to ensure you are both able and healthy enough to participate in this program.

Table Of Contents

Chapter 1: Understanding What Is Stress And How It Works 1

Chapter 2: Good Stress Versus Bad Stress 17

Chapter 3: Get It Out Of Your Mind 20

Chapter 4: Additional Ways To Reduce Your Stress For The Long Term 77

Chapter 5: Listen To Soothing Music 84

Chapter 6: How Stress Takes a Toll at the Brain and Behavior? 97

Chapter 7: Managing an Angry Brain ... 113

Chapter 8: Managing a Stressed Brain . 150

Chapter 9: Avert demanding situations from getting out of manipulate 174

Chapter 1: Understanding What Is Stress And How It Works

What exactly is strain? Psychologically talking, pressure has traditionally been described in strategies: stimulus-based totally totally or response-based totally. The stimulus-based definition of pressure indicates that strain comes from stress. The more the pressure, the greater strain you sense. We can all tolerate low stages of stress. Our brains may be quite poorly designed if we couldn't! But there can be a positive factor at the same time as the pressure will become too much, and your mind and frame start to undergo beneath the stress. While stimulus-primarily based totally pressure builds usually from outdoor stressors, it can then furthermore relate to inner stressors - a cumulative nature of pressure. In distinct phrases, the assemble-up of many tiny stresses may be sincerely as risky as one massive, stressful event (Butler, 1993).

The reaction-based definition of pressure, alternatively, shows that strain especially comes from horrific stimuli. This method focuses a good deal less on what causes the stress, and as an alternative specializes inside the severity of your frame's response to stressors. This definition explains why some element that is probably interesting or maybe trivial to as a minimum one person may be an intense deliver of tension for a few other person. The strategies in which the frame responds to pressure had been first divided into three measurable levels through manner of using Hans Selye within the Fifties. According to his research, the primary signal of strain in the frame is what he called an "alarm response" (Selye, 1956). Today, we generally call this the "fight-or-flight" response. Essentially, that is what takes place whilst your thoughts registers a capability danger. Whether that danger takes the shape of an oncoming train, a looming lease charge, or a gory scene in a horror movie, your thoughts and body will respond within the identical manner. Once a danger is detected, your thoughts starts to deliver one-of-a-type chemicals, and asks all of the structures of the body to be on immoderate-alert so you have the strength, power, and alertness you need to deal with the state of affairs. The stress response is, in concept, an first rate survival device. It transforms us into superbeings, and heightens all of our senses so as to combat chance. But in case you are in a consistent state of strain, then the stress response in no way is going away. Your body in no way has the risk to transport once more to its ordinary "relaxation-and-digest" state, in which you could relax.

If you preserve a combat-or-flight reaction extended sufficient, your frame is going into the second degree of strain, what Selye calls "resistance" (1956). In this degree, your thoughts is in struggle with itself. Your conscious thoughts is privy to which you are not in on the spot chance, but your subconscious thoughts isn't always satisfied. Unfortunately, it's the subconscious thoughts that triggers and subdues the stress response. You can be in a position to influence yourself that the entirety is fantastic, but it takes masses more than electricity of will to steer your body. This is the extent in which you start to cope with your strain a good way to relieve it. But there are healthy and terrible techniques to address stress. If we aren't virtually privy to what happens internal our body, we are able to without troubles fall into lousy coping strategies like anger, manipulation, or avoidance. If this resistance degree continues for too lengthy, your frame will input the 0.33 degree, what Selye calls "disintegrate" or "exhaustion" (1956). It is at this detail which you begin to see physical or intellectual health troubles appear, which may be without delay related to your pressure.

We realize now that every definitions of stimulus-based totally and response-based absolutely strain are beneficial and essential. It can be very critical to recognise in which your stress is coming from, but it is also important to recognize why you respond in your stressors the way which you do. Your person, lifestyles instances, past traumas, and on occasion your genetics all combine to decide what pressures purpose you to feel pressure and the techniques you glaringly reap for to cope with your stressors.

Stress is depending on factors: the needs being positioned on you via the scenario, and the sources that you want to meet the ones needs (Butler, 1993). If the state of affairs asks you to do extra than you're capable of, then you definitely definately start to revel in stress. The capture, but, is that needs and assets aren't objective phrases. Unfortunately, stress is not based in fact, pressure is based totally in the manner you for my part perceive the state of affairs. Your thoughts, attitudes, ideals, and fantasies all combine to create a completely particular know-how of your self and your state of affairs. If you accept as true with that you aren't capable of meet a undertaking, or not capable sufficient to effectively navigate a state of affairs, then you'll start to revel in pressure. This occurs even if your perception is unfounded or truely unfaithful. Stress, then, may be seen as a shape of relationship. A courting among you and the area round you. Stress arises at the same time as some issue for your lifestyles, whether or not or not or not it's some other individual, a bill, or a workload, drains you of all your assets and consequently places you in risk. The hazard of unemployment, divorce, or the incapacity to provide an wonderful domestic to your children are all very actual situations that might motive your body's pressure responses. It need to also be the threat of bodily hazard, like exhaustion.

Because stress is prepared the manner you recognize a situation, and not simply the state of affairs itself, there are as many different types of stressors as there are human beings within the worldwide. What makes you shrivel up internal with dread should possibly seem mundane or stupid to a person else. Something that makes you experience excited, or projects that you experience going for walks on, might also set some other's teeth on side. There's no such detail, then, as a stressor that's "not a big deal." If the situation motives you to feel strain, then it's a huge deal to you. It doesn't make you susceptible or incapable, it's clearly part of who you are. The answer isn't to "stop" feeling confused approximately a few thing, as a substitute, the solution is to determine out what it's miles approximately that state of affairs that is causing you to experience pressured. Anxiety and stress recommend that a few issue approximately the situation inside the front of you feels threatening. For a few detail purpose, you sense like you don't have the time, strength, intelligence, or budget to cope with the mission in the front of you. That is the sensation that we name "stress," and that is what we want to realize inside ourselves.

How Stress Affects the Brain

Ceaseless Stress Increases Mental Illness

In an exam allotted in Molecular Psychiatry, professionals discovered that constant strain brings about lengthy-haul adjustments inside the cerebrum. These changes, they recommend, may likely assist make clear why the individuals who enjoy ceaseless pressure are moreover extra willing to mind-set and uneasiness issues in some time at some stage in normal lifestyles.

Stress performs a huge role in inflicting highbrow problems, which incorporates sorrow and precise enthusiastic problems. Specialists from the University of California—Berkeley performed out a progression of trials taking a gander at the effect of constant weight on the cerebrum. They found that such stress makes extra myelin-developing cells, but plenty much less neurons than regular. The aftereffect of this disturbance is an abundance of myelin in specific regions of the thoughts, which meddles with the state of affairs and parity of correspondence. The analysts positioned that stress can likewise affect the mind's hippocampus.

Stress Changes the Brain's Structure

The aftereffects of examinations thru professionals from the University of California—Berkeley uncovered that interminable pressure can spark off prolonged haul adjustments inside the form and capability of the thoughts.

The mind is made from neurons and backing cells (darkish problem), which may be used for dynamic and essential wondering. Yet, the mind furthermore incorporates what's known as white problem, this is created from the apparent multitude of axons that interface with one-of-a-type locales of the cerebrum to carry facts.

White trouble is so named because of the greasy, white sheath referred to as myelin that encompasses the axons that accelerate the electric symptoms and signs and signs and symptoms used to convey facts in a few unspecified time inside the destiny of the thoughts.

The overproduction of myelin that the specialists noticed due to the nearness of interminable strain doesn't virtually result in a short exchange to be determined amongst white and dim trouble—it could likewise spark off enduring changes in the cerebrum's shape.

Specialists and analysts have in recent times visible that humans experiencing located up-horrendous pressure difficulty have thoughts irregularities remembering dark and white issues.

Clinician Daniela Kaufer, the expert within the again of those examinations, recommends that not all stress affects the thoughts and neural systems in addition. There is a sort of strain that encourages you to perform well no matter a check, supporting with wiring the thoughts in a pleasing manner, prompting more grounded systems and in addition prominent flexibility.

Ceaseless fear, however, can set off masses of issues. You're developing a cerebrum that is each hard or in reality helpless in opposition to highbrow infection, in view of the designing of white problem you get right off the bat all through ordinary life, clarified Kaufer.

Stress Kills Brain Cells

In an research led via the usage of specialists from the Rosalind Franklin University of Medicine and Science, analysts located that a lonely socially-stressing event may additionally want to murder new neurons in the cerebrum's hippocampus.

The hippocampus is one of the locales of the cerebrum vigorously associated with reminiscence, feeling, and studying. It is likewise one of the territories of the cerebrum wherein neurogenesis, or the affiliation of recent synapses, takes region in the course of life.

In exams, the exam corporation set younger rodents in a pen with extra seasoned rodents for a time of 20 minutes. The greater younger rodent grow to be then uncovered to animosity from the extra skilled occupants of the confine. Later evaluation of the younger rodents located that that they had cortisol tiers as an lousy lot as a couple of instances higher than that of rodents who had now not encountered an frightening social enjoy.

Further evaluation exposed that at the equal time as the more youthful rodents set under stress had produced comparable variety of latest neurons due to the fact the folks who had not encountered the concern, there has been a checked decrease in the amount of nerve cells seven days after the truth. While strain may not appear to impact the association of latest neurons, it impacts whether or not or no longer or no longer the ones cells go through. So, strain can execute synapses, but is there a few issue need to be feasible to limit the harming effect of strain?

Stress Shrinks the Brain

Stress can spark off shrinkage in zones of the mind associated with the rule of feelings, digestion, and memory.

While humans regularly associate awful outcomes to sudden, notable strain made by way of existence converting events, (for instance, a cataclysmic occasion, car collision, passing of a chum or family member), scientists in fact suggest that it's far the ordinary strain that we as a whole seem to confront that, after some time, can upload to a good sized scope of intellectual issues.

In one examination, analysts from Yale University took a gander at 100 sound members who gave information about the frightening sports activities in their lives. The specialists noticed that presentation to stretch, even ongoing stress, brought about the mind to cut back inside the prefrontal cortex, a locale of the cerebrum connected to such things as poise and emotions.

Ceaseless, normal strain seemed to have little effect on cerebrum quantity all by myself but can also additionally make human beings more helpless towards thoughts shrinkage at the same time as they're faced with great, horrible stressors. The growth of existence occasions which is probably stressing may additionally moreover moreover make it tougher for those people to control future strain, specially if the subsequent inquiring for event requires effortful control, feeling guiding principle, or coordinated social managing to defeat it, clarified the examination's lead writer, Emily Ansell.

Various sorts of pressure have an effect at the thoughts in numerous manners. Ongoing distressing sports (paintings misfortune, fender bender) effect passionate mindfulness. Horrible accidents (passing of a friend or family member, genuine ailment) significantly have an effect on disposition focuses.

Stress Hurts Your Memory

In the event that you have at any element tried to remember the subtleties of an ugly occasion, you're most likely conscious that, every so often, strain can motive sports to be tough to keep in thoughts. Indeed, even reasonably minor pressure can right away affect your memory, as an example, seeking to do not forget where your automobile keys are or wherein you left your folder case when you aren't on time for paintings.

One 2012 studies discovered that incessant strain negatively affects what is called spatial memory. This is the reminiscence that data facts in your spatial orientation and environment. A modern file exposed that substantial levels of the pressure hormone cortisol have been associated with brief memory decreases in greater seasoned rodents.

The popular effect of stress on memory depends on different factors, considered one in every of it is timing. Various investigations have showed that after pressure happens preceding getting to know, reminiscence is fantastically affected and it is able to be upgraded thru a memory consolidation.

Then yet again, strain has been appeared to avoid memory recuperation. For instance, professionals have continuously indicated that presentation to stretch certainly in advance than a memory protection test activates dwindled execution in every human and creature topics.

While strain is actually some component that can not be prevented in existence, specialists do get preserve of that thru seeing exactly how and why stress influences the cerebrum, they can choose out up understanding into forestalling or in any occasion, solving a part of the damage stress brings. For instance, some specialists endorse that such examination need to are on the lookout for for to enhance medicinal capsules intended to forestall the terrible impacts of pressure on the mind.

Chapter 2: Good Stress Versus Bad Stress

Good strain, moreover known as eustress, is the strain felt even as we get excited. It makes our pulse to rush up and the hormones to surge. When we pass on a number one date, journey the curler coaster, or compete for selling, we sense this stress. This shape of suitable strain has many incentives, it makes us whole of strength and excitement in existence.

The traits of real pressure are as follows:

- It enables beautify general typical overall performance
- It motivates, focuses power.
- It has a experience of satisfaction.
- Is seen as inner our coping talents.
- It is short-time period.

On the alternative hand, horrible stress is the alternative of excellent strain. It's the stress that takes on a top notch mind-set. A mindset that is going into the negatives. When an individual has awful pressure, they'll often reflectively accomplice pressure with terrible topics from the beyond. Some will revel in like they was first rate before it happened; like it should no longer have occurred to them. Bad pressure can also occur because of an inconvenience or something that interrupts the ordinary time desk. It's called, 'horrible pressure' due to the truth the way it affects you isn't top; it feels one-of-a-kind. Life is disturbing while you get careworn approximately little topics that make life greater hard than they must. But it is pinnacle to be privy to it. Because regardless of in that you pass on this worldwide, horrible pressure will constantly find you. You can't keep away from it.

Some of the traits of horrible stress include:

- It has an unpleasant feeling.

- It creates concern or anxiety.

- It is visible as outside of our coping talents.

- It can bring about bodily and intellectual troubles.

- It declines ordinary overall performance.
- It can be quick- or prolonged-time period.

Chapter 3: Get It Out Of Your Mind

Step 1 - Jot It Down

Using a mag for self-improvement is one of the exquisite methods to benefit greater strength of mind. I have for my part used a magazine to alleviate strain and it works. Here is the manner it passed off.

In this international, pressure is inevitable however it's miles critical the manner you manipulate it. Write down a few component you enjoy like; it may be your feelings, someone's moves or perhaps a few incidents. Write down your mind, do not determine them, actually permit it waft out. Once you get commenced on this, you are first-rate to feel a weight off your chest. Things which had been bothering you'll slowly subside just like ink on pages. It is set up that if we permit subjects out on paper, we revel in consolation. It's the first rate resource you can find out. I am quite wonderful that you have seen people write their emotions down and in case you've observed, they continuously regarded to be calmer and happier.

If you have got were given were given a topic of maximum hassle, a difficulty that has been tormenting your thoughts for a long time and if you have been now not capable of get a grip over it, the best way to deal with it is by means of the usage of way of writing. In existence, we spend masses on matters so we are capable of feel satisfied, obtain achievement and suit on this crazy global. In the face of all this, little or no interest is given to at least one in every of our most critical organs, the thoughts. It's right that the frame is what you can sense, but it's miles simplest the mind that permits us to revel in. If your mind is wholesome, you'll be healthy; in case your thoughts is at peace, you may be at peace. But are not absolutely everyone responsible of ignoring this fact? Well, we have a propensity to bear in mind that we're capable of type out the messes in our existence by using the usage of our frame, and we turn to such approach as capsules, alcohol and such to take away the pain. Is that in truth the proper manner to transport about it? Of route not, for that would make you relying on those subjects all the time. You want to learn how to take one step at a time, you need to try and kind subjects out by using converting the way you be aware them, simplest then will you be capable of parent out the right manner to address them. Is it going to be an easy road? There's a possibility of difficulties, however you want to try, and you have to attempt to make it the terrific that it could ever be.

The excellent issue about journaling is that it does not rate you a dime, I suggest, you best want to apply the paper that you find out for your own family. I apprehend that subjects are not as correct as they appear nearly about preserving a journal due to the fact every time I try to write I experience that sure part of my thoughts is telling me it is a waste of time. But guess what, that a part of my thoughts became wrong, like I said, that may be a modern manner of coping with our problems. This is with out value, it's why I locate it irresistible lots. And the sort of manner is generally going to be an efficient way of attaining you. Get the magazine, write your issues, thoughts and your problems, and whilst you're completed, positioned them into the magazine. Set apart a while each day to take a look at through the mag and decide for your self whether or not or no longer the mind do or do now not seem as suitable as you felt them at the begin. Keep it to 2 pages at a time, have a look at them then placed away. Don't go away behind any unfastened ends because of the fact this is in which the pressure starts offevolved to creep in.

There is every other first rate element approximately writing, it gives you a feel of introspection. After writing my troubles and mind, it generally allows me to parent out in which exactly the problem is and as quickly as I am capable of do that then I can see the manner out. But this isn't for surely absolutely everyone. Let's face it, we are all terrific and so are our minds. That's why I cannot say that this mag aspect will artwork right away to your problem too, however it truely doesn't harm to try. You don't have some thing to lose. And I wager that is only a tip, a tip that could be a high-quality leap in your lifestyles towards a happier life. You had been compelled, now you may now not be careworn. Now you will enhance and it will likely be so easy!

Go earlier and write down your emotions in your mag, it will assist.

Step 2 - Learn To Say 'No'

Don't try to be all people's hero at artwork. Many people can also depend on your abilties and goodwill to hold their day, however although it makes you enjoy pinnacle to be the individual humans turn to of their hour of want, be careful no longer to place yourself in a function in which human beings will count on which you'll drop the whole lot to help them with their troubles. You want to examine to say "no." You don't need to be imply approximately it but be excellent and company. A easy statement will do: "I'm sorry, but I actually can't help you proper now. I'll fortunately help you first in the morning."

To lessen your very personal strain and honestly have right paintings-life stability, you need to spend extra of it gradual and power focusing in your own dreams and the goals of your family.

If you've have been given masses of tough paintings to do however your boss offers you more duties, don't artwork your self right into a frenzy, specially in case you recognize it's an unfair expectation. Don't torture yourself or jeopardize your fitness due to the fact you stated "high-quality" to some thing you shouldn't have. Have the self notion and self-respect to move and talk to your boss. Point out that the mission cannot be finished thru the usage of one person, and that you could't do it till a few unique colleague is assigned to assist. In this example, pronouncing "no" no longer quality protects you from capability burnout but additionally shows your professionalism.

Too many social sports can overload you, too, and you want to be for the reason that you may't be in locations right away. Rushing from one event to the subsequent may be tremendously annoying, so you need to determine which sports activities sports to mention "yes" to and which to mention "no" to. If you discover that you are pronouncing "sure" to property you don't actually need to do, that take you far from your family, or that causes you strain, you want to get cushty with declining invitations without guilt or disgrace. If your work pals ask you to go out to dinner with them however you may alternatively definitely spend time collectively along with your big exclusive, pronouncing, "no, thanks," is a fantastically lower priced reaction.

Being more aware about "no" may even help you avoid burning out from overwork. You can with out difficulty overstretch your self by means of the usage of manner of taking over greater requests than you could contend with, after which you need to come up with a final-minute excuse for the stuff you've dedicated to doing. A "no" permit you to avoid conditions that pressure you out. The extra stress you experience from having to constantly clean up unique people's messes, the higher the risk that you'll moreover overextend yourself via promising too many things to too many human beings.

When you're able to say "no" to humans for your very own phrases on occasion, you could moreover sense higher approximately yourself, to be able to in addition distance you from the guilt and self-punishment you could experience for not doing what others ask from you. Then, you'll feel extra assured in yourself and your options and you'll moreover sense an entire lot much less strain to continuously be given requests.

When you are making the choice to get worried with special humans, you may face an entire lot of conflicting requests. You'll meet with one-of-a-kind humans on brilliant activities and you'll get used to assisting every of them with their problems. But similar to in the actual worldwide, the ones human beings will normally now not be there to rely upon for the lengthy-time period. Another man or woman's needs and problems aren't nearly as critical as yours, and also you need to have the capability to mention "no" with out being judged.

It's proper that many exceptional people may additionally desire that they may say no to every person as well. If you find out yourself announcing "yes" to every body, you'll turn out to be in a normal united states of america of being overwhelmed. You will feel trapped via the individuals who rely on you to solve their issues, and you may no longer be able to waft on collectively collectively with your very own goals or promises.

Deciding to say "no" to human beings and searching after your self is tough only due to the fact you have been conditioned to say positive to the whole thing. Making the selection to mention "no" to different human beings isn't always a problem, but it does take exercising. You want to set a few ground regulations for your self, despite the fact that, so you received't get too wrapped up in what wonderful human beings want you to do.

You have to make your very very own choices without worrying about how others will react to what you assert. You ought to set your priorities and also you want to make sure that you're not overextending yourself. It's really k to show down a request, and it's without a doubt ok to say "no" to human beings.

Knowing how to mention "no" might also even help you discover ways to begin announcing "no" to dangerous behavior. We all have horrific behavior that we will do without, and we need to mention "no" to them via developing our very personal healthful behavior with a purpose to create a huge distinction for your lifestyles. When you've got got your private behavior, you will be better able to assert yourself, and your new behavior will include saying "no" to those risky conduct. For instance, if you're not the type of individual who enjoys consuming alcohol, and also you discover your self associating that preference with people who constantly ask you to join them, you then should learn the way to mention "no."

Many human beings will assume that you can say "sure" sincerely because of the fact you're similar to those people. But you must in no manner be that shape of character. If you need to create healthy behavior, then you definately ought to mention "no" to ingesting alcohol. By saying "no" to other human beings's dreams for you, you can start to analyze the manner to say "no" to your private conduct that you don't virtually enjoy or need. This will will let you create new momentum for yourself and begin to live the existence which you expected for yourself.

The secret's to mention "no" best to matters that you don't want to your lifestyles. You don't want to have risky conduct, and also you don't want human beings for your life who make horrible options that negatively have an impact on you.

The largest way to react to unstable behavior is to mention "no" to the folks who make the ones behavior take place. Say "no" to bad conduct with the aid of pronouncing "no" to the people who invite you to those dangerous sports. You furthermore want to keep in mind that each awful preference that you make can also have a terrible impact in your destiny. There are sure people on your lifestyles who supply you down, and you need to say "no" and surrender those relationships.

Step 3 - Make Time For Play

Your life shouldn't sincerely be just about work (housework protected). It's very vital which you make time to do things that you very well revel in. Make time for romancing, traveling, going to pastime activities, going to the theater, or gambling loopy rides at enjoyment parks. The assets you do for herbal leisure are a part of who you're. Don't lose your fun thing actually due to the fact your days are packed with all the duties of being a expert. Going off and simply performing some thing for the fun of it is able to be a remarkable way to alleviate stress and feel correct. When you circulate lower back to art work, you may be higher ready to deal with some thing strain is thrown your way due to the reality that you may shake it off by manner of the usage of making time for play.

The first benefit of play is that it allows us adapt to lifestyles. Play lets in children and extra youthful human beings increase coping techniques for later lifestyles. When play and artwork become merged right proper right into a ordinary ordinary, one becomes not able to conform as it should be to more tough worrying situations. By adapting to demanding situations, play teaches the ordinary person the manner to cope with sudden and vital problems.

Secondly, play fosters creativity because it continues the individual thinking about opportunities in region of questioning in a restrained way. If one in no manner gets outdoor of the "useful" education of wondering, one by no means receives to the current thoughts. In a few organizations, gambling has turn out to be a supply of recent products. These businesses rate creativity and imagination.

Thirdly, the praise one receives from play lets in to provide the individual a experience of identification. Many humans start to lose their revel in of who they may be after they prevent gambling. Many people artwork really to get coins to shop for cloth possessions for which they have got little use. The time spent on paintings takes up maximum of their time, leaving no unfastened time for themselves to play. The alienation from themselves accumulates.

Fourthly, play can increase and preserve proper relationships. Play allows shape friendships. When humans do no longer play and make bigger their skills, they may skip over out on many opportunities to shape relationships. There are hundreds of possibilities to socialise with people that play numerous sports activities sports, but at the same time as that possibility is unnoticed, relationships can not be advanced. Conversely, as gambling develops people's capabilities, they're capable of create and hold relationships due to this.

Playing is also beneficial in relieving stress due to the fact play derives from the man or woman's preference for manage over their environment, it permits in bringing stability and order to as a minimum one's life. This relieves strain because it gives the character once more their freedom of choice.

Playing furthermore allows in relieving stress at domestic. Parents can unfastened themselves from a number of the problems furnished within the place of job that make paintings a each day war. They can discover ways to lighten up and characteristic fun with their kids all once more. By permitting one's kids to play and boom, parents also can grow to be extra comfortable at home.

In summary, play is beneficial in that it lets in cast off the stress and isolation of difficult paintings.

Section 2 - Immediate Ways To Radically Reduce Your Stress

Step 4 - Exercise

It's essential for prolonged-time period strain sufferers to get regular exercising, particularly if their existence require hours of the use of or sitting at a table all day prolonged. You may also moreover have grow to be acquainted with sitting despite the fact that for a long term on prevent, however your body want and desires to be energetic on a each day basis, and in case you don't comply, your frame will begin to item and show uncomfortable signs and symptoms and symptoms and signs and signs and symptoms and signs of strain that first-rate movement can remedy.

Health is wealth, they will be pronouncing, and also you need to are looking for to preserve yourself within the top notch possible country of health. You can kick away pressure and stay in suitable shape physical and mentally with the useful aid of exercise often. Make a addiction of exercising each day. If you're making a dependancy of waking up early, you may have sufficient time to meditate and exercising. If you do not have enough time to exercise sufficiently inside the mornings, you may generally do it within the night time time. You want to certainly find out a way to artwork it into your day. Many humans choose out to get their workout out of the manner first hassle inside the morning. This allows you revel in better and further energized, and then later inside the day, you received't need to be considering carving out time to exercise. Instead, you could attention at the subjects that need to get completed. Exercising first problem inside the morning can also help sharpen intellectual readability, making you greater effective in the direction of the day. Regular exercising can be very useful and you want to get concerned.

Exercise and excessive-electricity sports sports sports activities activities are quite effective close to liberating tension. You want to be careful not to overexert your self, however sweating it out in some unspecified time inside the destiny of an notable exercising will deliver prolonged-time period stress a run for its cash.

Good sporting sports for stress discount embody:

- Aerobics
- Running
- Jogging
- Roller Skating
- Dancing
- Swimming
- Tennis
- Cycling

If you need to enjoy right now pressure-release, you need to get your frame transferring and your coronary heart pumping.

Yoga is every one-of-a-type form of exercising that allow you to lessen your extended-time period strain. Most human beings expect yoga may be very peaceful, however it does embody some of physical movements. Some sorts of yoga can also moreover even integrate aerobic workout or weights for a nicely-rounded art work-out. Further, yoga is a relaxing and truely effective thoughts-body hobby that releases tension via posture bodily video video video video games, which is probably mixed with deep respiratory strategies.

Studies in current years advise the super importance of physical interest, now not best in preserving your health (improving cardiovascular staying energy, and strengthening the neural tool, the skeleton, and muscle organizations), but additionally in improving the mind and its talents.

Researchers in the region maintain that strenuous workout allows the cognitive improvement of our brains.

How does bodily interest have an effect on cognitive development? Exercise is critical for thoughts improvement and it impacts its improvement in masses of techniques, which encompass: superior oxygen intake, expanded secretion of neurotransmitters, and prolonged secretion of neurotrophins.

During exercise, oxygen consumption and blood flow increase. This permits oxygen and blood to circulate the muscle tissues, collectively with the mind. In this manner it have become determined that new blood vessels are created in a way called angiogenesis inside the thoughts.

The oxygen uptake inside the direction of workout improves the blood go together with the go with the flow in regions of the thoughts which may be essential for cognitive duties.

A 2d mechanism allows bodily hobby to growth ranges of neurotransmitters, collectively with serotonin and norepinephrine. This increase of neurotransmitters allows the processing of records in the mind. A massive quantity of those substances allows for additonal inexperienced "wiring" of the neuronal community within the thoughts, making communique and transmission of the chemical messages many of the numerous nerve cells and the most effective-of-a-type areas of the mind greater inexperienced.

Over time, physical workout results in mind schooling, because of this that that that the massive sort of thoughts connections will boom and so will its function.

The 0.33 mechanism reasons an boom in secretion of neurotrophins in the direction of physical exercising. Neurotrophins are the proteins responsible for thoughts tissue and are quite important in generating the materials that nerve cells want in the long run of our young humans development.

The characteristic of neurotrophins is also to maintain mind cells, and to ensure their survival at an older age at the equal time because the charge of thoughts mobile manufacturing is reducing. It has been confirmed that however the reality that the fee of producing decreases as we age, there are however areas of the thoughts wherein new nerve cells are developing.

The mechanism is chargeable for this works, among extraordinary subjects, through neurotrophins. It follows that a better secretion of those materials will no longer simplest help keep modern-day-day mind cells, however they may furthermore stimulate the appearance of latest cells in later age.

The thoughts of historical humankind required bodily hobby not awesome to keep off chance, but furthermore to conform as human beings. The human thoughts these days moreover calls for bodily interest.

Although human beings in recent times now not frequently should physical get away from danger, they do want talents which includes choice-making at an powerful tempo, and statistics garage to constantly cope with the numerous stimuli in their environment.

It has been borne out that oldsters which can be bodily lively all their lives furthermore have true cognitive skills. Some mother and father experience we've were given got a real want for bodily interest, that it's miles a name for of our mind.

But what approximately folks that don't enjoy the want? The solution probably lies in our genetics. Research in this case is ongoing every day and the relevant genes have not all began to had been really mapped, but in my estimation we're able to quick be able to recognize the genetic mapping that makes some of us want bodily hobby and others who're certainly not interested in it.

Genetic studies can assist the "sofa potatoes amongst us." In my experience, you in fact should get commenced out out out, slowly in advance than everything, and in a managed manner. In this way, the mechanisms we defined earlier will come into play and through the years, our brains will extend a need for a more quantity of those substances.

The cycle will start to feed upon itself and could keep us going with exercise.

Step 5 - Mindfulness

I understand that many readers will need to get right now to an information of the manner mindfulness can help and the manner they may be able to encompass it into their lives with consequences, so I will no longer deliver an in-depth information of mindfulness. This is a practical e-book entire of sensible physical sports sports activities, recommendations, and techniques to gather into your every day lifestyles.

Mindfulness isn't an esoteric or spiritual workout (irrespective of the reality that it could be if that is a part of someone's perception tool). Mindfulness has its roots in non secular ideals and practices. What I am providing in this e-book are strategies that have been tested to paintings.

One of the remarkable factors of mindfulness is that it can be practiced pretty loads everywhere with minimum try to no detail consequences. Once you have got got determined out the strategies, it's far free. It is suitable for human beings of all ranges of health, age, electricity, and backgrounds.

Despite what a few people would possibly possibly probably expect, in truth anybody can be aware. I choice to provide you the steerage and assist you may want to make certain mindfulness will become 2d nature to your every day lifestyles. I want to help you create a middle of peace and contentment for your inner-most being that can't be ruffled thru the worrying conditions and stressors of every day life.

Mindfulness lets in us to be aware of our subjective perceptions and views. This reputation can help deliver us insights into searching at our reality otherwise. These insights can help us re-frame how we experience lifestyles. This altered interest can assist ease and soothe the pain and terror of panic and strain.

Mindfulness gives us a hard and rapid of self-soothing tool that make our annoying opinions an entire lot a good buy masses less worrying.

Attitude of Mindfulness

Many of the attitudes beneficial useful resource each precise and will almost be interchangeable; the attitudes are all elements of the same gemstone of mindfulness.

The term mindfulness is a misnomer. What we're doing on the identical time as we exercise mindfulness is endeavoring to free the self from the thoughts. Our minds control how we live in the ones modern-day-day instances.

In Asian languages, the terms 'mind' and 'coronary coronary coronary coronary heart' are used interchangeably. Therefore, mindfulness might be understood as 'heartfulness'. This makes masses of intuitive experience. By consciously integrating attitudes together with those listed beneath, we're operating towards 'heartfulness'. This connects us with others.

We can notable take a look at our emotional fitness in relationships with others. We can not stay on our meditation cushion all of the time. We need to get off the cushion and take our 'heartfulness' out into the area. The attitudes are the tool we're able to use to workout in the actual worldwide. Practicing (and because of this sometimes failing at) the ones attitudes is like every different functionality, we need to exercise it. We can studies from our errors and flow into on. Such efforts will enhance us out of the jail of terrible self-belief that could feed tension and strain. By searching outward with natural reasons and intentions, we can navigate thru life's demanding conditions with extra serenity and intellectual peace.

Closing the Expectation Gap

The extra we are capable of embody the ones attitudes in how we perform in the worldwide, in relationships with ourselves and others, mindfulness becomes an lousy lot much less about a exercise and in addition approximately who we are. It's a preference we're capable of make every morning: do I want to be extra compassionate, affected person, present, inclined, accepting, forgiving, and thankful? By choosing the direction of mindfulness/heartfulness, we're final the distance amongst what we expect and what's. The hole is the no-man's-land of anxiety and suffering. By final the gap, we're able to stay a life of which means that that that that, depth, and peace.

Compassion

Many people hold in thoughts compassion as an emotion or a revel in. It is greater of a tool. The first step is to be present. Be positioned on your personal life; revel in actually what goes on in someone second.

The next diploma of compassion is being in-song with the alternative individual, feeling empathy and human identity. To illustrate this trouble, the Chinese man or woman for listening includes five elements: the ears, the eyes, you, me, and coronary coronary coronary coronary heart. This is a visible reminder of strategies we are capable of pay hobby actively to others, through using attractive not really the ears and eyes, however moreover connecting with the coronary coronary coronary heart. The act of being completely present and in music with the opportunity individual is a mindfulness exercise in compassion.

The final diploma of the manner is wishing the super for that individual or proceeding to alleviate their struggling. This can be a realistic motion or if we cannot take a realistic step, we want to make a sincere choice that their suffering is alleviated.

Compassion reminds us of the deep bond we've got were given were given with others. Einstein stated this even as he talked about the self-imposed prisons of questioning we're separate. He cautioned people to: 'Widen our circle of compassion to embody all living subjects.'

Acceptance

This is an active technique of choosing to certainly accept what is going on within the gift second. We don't want to find it irresistible or stress ourselves to revel in it.

Make location to allow for some detail situation or revel in it is. We can plan to cast off ourselves from an unwanted existence scenario. Having a plan can help ease the unfastened-floating anxiety of the unknown. We will speak approximately planning later inside the e-book.

The next degree is letting go along with the go together with the waft of the consequences, letting the plan unfold. We need to keep away from playing highbrow movies in our head of the way topics need to unfold. Just due to the truth you want something to take area, it is easy to really acquire as proper with that this is how topics need to be, and we grow to be unhappy if life chooses a amazing very last consequences. If you allow go together with the flow of the consequences, you are more able to roll with life's unsightly surprises, so you don't get damage. Moreover, life's complete of surprises. If you aren't wedded to a first rate final results, you could see while lifestyles is handing you an surprising possibility and take whole gain of that.

Acceptance isn't resignation. You can take powerful motion. Taking effective motion is higher than staying stuck in terrible motion together with feeling or appearing irritated, worried, and irritated. When we take transport of the triumphing second, we allow for brought possibilities inside the scenario and a lighter power of preference, possibility, and desire.

Letting Go

Powerful emotions inclusive of worry, anxiety, resentment, and anger can enjoy almost no longer viable to permit waft of. Resentment or anger, mainly if it looks as if righteous anger, can skip round and round in our heads, burning up right electricity like a grasping flame. Holding proper away to resentment has been likened to consuming poison and hoping the other man or woman dies. Resentment will only damage you and no character else.

Practicing tolerance, splendor, and compassion with a scenario that conjures up anger, worry or resentment can help. Taking the character or state of affairs from your head and into your coronary coronary heart can also additionally artwork.

In practical terms, because of this letting the angry/concerned/worried/envious mind go with the flow. Instead of ruminating on beyond injustices/fears/what-ifs/what could have been and so forth. Focus on your coronary coronary heart and channel the emotional strength of the situation a protracted way from the top and into the coronary coronary coronary coronary heart.

In this manner, you are acknowledging how important this case is or has been to you. You aren't disregarding it; you're redirecting it to an area in which you'll be a first rate deal a good deal less mentally thru it.

In addition, trusting your coronary heart with this man or woman or scenario will melt the harshness, unhappiness, judgment or anger that would surround the situation. Above all, gather that letting flow is a manner. Sometimes it's a extended device. There is not commonly a as fast as and for all dramatic incidence.

We can discover that we permit one problem pass, and then some component else pops up. That's being human. Keep working on letting drift as a continual paintings in development.

Non-Striving

That is sailing with the wind in location of rowing furiously in opposition to it. We may moreover want to have a plan, a holiday spot, however we don't want to push so difficult. We can take movement and the stairs to get to the vacation spot, however we don't need to overstretch or overwork and pressure ourselves out. It is prepared yielding, in vicinity of opposing the go together with the flow of existence. You can first-class experience the float of life in the gift second. In martial arts, a key concept is to yield to triumph over. Opposition and stress create competition and pressure.

Non-Judging

When I speak approximately judging I propose the tough judgement that has undertones of awful criticism, blame, and shame. We can use our discretion and intelligence to determine that a scenario or character won't be strong for us. We can use our mind to offer beneficial feedback on a bit of difficult art work or a challenge to help beautify it or expand talents.

In relating to others, non-judging is part of beauty and compassion. If we're with a person, we take transport of them in truth as they may be at that 2nd. We don't get hung up on what we don't like or reputation on elements in their man or woman or look we assume they need to change.

You are gift with them, within the proper proper right here and now, absolutely as they may be. This includes your self.

If we must loose ourselves up from the concern of our very personal or simply certainly one of a kind people's choices, endure in thoughts how free you'll be to be whoever and some detail you need. Fear of numerous people's awful opinion dad and mom can paralyze us; it limits growth and contemporary undertaking.

By all technique, ask for and take shipping of comments, but unsolicited critiques are the organisation of severa humans. Stay in the middle of your very very very very own existence and don't get too stuck up within the options of others.

Be aware about your personal 'inner critic' and don't get worried in harsh self-options—see them as in truth 'thoughts' and allow them to transport.

Gratitude

Appreciation is acknowledging the charge of some issue. Being thankful is a few element you could experience and do. Look spherical and admire the whole thing you've got from the maximum number one life essential to the most fairly-present day gadgets or systems. Relatively talking, we're able to stay a lifestyles that for our forbearers may be considered a lifestyles of ease and comfort. As with most of those attitudes, gratitude is a device.

Be present, understand what you experience all spherical you, and be thankful. By filling our hearts and minds with mind of gratitude and appreciation we are filling up intellectual and emotional location that might be complete of negativity, worry, tension, and resentment.

Gratitude is strong, mainly on the identical time as you enjoy down. If you are having an unpleasant day, or likely going through a difficult time on your lifestyles, you can enjoy which you do not have some thing to be pleased about. But there may be constantly some element. If you ruminate on the negatives on your lifestyles, you could possibly definitely discover more negativity.

Gratitude breaks the terrible downward spiral.

Willingness

If any of these attitudes enjoy past you inside the advise time, absolutely be willing to permit them to into your popularity.

Most of them are part of a manner. Keep an open and curious thoughts and be willing to attempt out some mind. Play approximately with the thoughts, strive being attentive to a guided meditation, reflecting on an attitude, journaling about it or exercising specializing in an thoughts-set as you skip approximately your every day lifestyles and actually see what takes place.

Be open to opportunities.

Be inclined to trade and word your lifestyles situation and who you're in a completely precise slight.

Patience

Adopting those attitudes will take time and exercise. Just do what you can, a touch every day. Consistency is essential. All the attitudes emerge as much less complicated to don't forget and to apply to your lifestyles on the same time as you're honestly placed in every 2d.

MEDITATION

One of the top notch strategies to control your thoughts and body at the same time as growing more strength of thoughts is to workout meditation on a every day basis. You don't need to make an entire-blown ritual, complete with incense sticks, candles and chimes ringing within the statistics. Meditate every time and everywhere you're snug.

The concept is to be more conscious and practical of your thoughts and movements. It is a incredible manner to direct your thoughts and thoughts in a disciplined manner. The idea is to comb away the cobwebs of horrible mind that take over our mind periodically.

Research has showed that our success is right now impacted via our internal energy of will and stress. A everyday and regular meditation workout can appreciably maximize your power of mind, treatment, and energy of will.

We all crave immediately gratification in a few unspecified time in the destiny or the opportunity without worrying approximately the ramifications or consequences of it. It is like craving a "recovery." In the ecstasy of immediately gratification, lengthy-term goals turn out to be fuzzy. There's little guilt or remorse on the equal time as you bear in mind you studied of immediately rewards. For instance, a difficult and speedy of buddies shows you be part of them for an extended weekend journey if you have an vital meeting springing up on Monday. The temptation of going for a relaxing tour over a monotonous assembly at art work can be immoderate.

I recommend you'd as an possibility be sitting on a mountain cabin partying together collectively together with your buddies than sitting within the path of a humdrum boss and co-employees. However, is skipping paintings contributing in your purpose of a vending or getting a better pay or moving to a higher organization? Once you've completed your restore, you may plunge into the same vintage guilt and regret of getting not noted an essential day at paintings. Does it make you experience appropriate approximately the holiday you've certainly loved?

Meditation prevents you from taking such impulsive, warmth of the right away and negative alternatives. How approximately consuming a bag of chips on the identical time as you're on a healthy eating plan? Or smoking when you have decided to get rid of intake of nicotine all of the time? When you meditate, you are plenty an awful lot a good deal much less possibly to make the ones "for the immediate" selections and maintain in thoughts prolonged-time period ramifications of every preference.

Duke University scientists studied the brains of 37 those who were eating regimen on the identical time as they were showed photos of severa tempting components. The studies located out that the mind's dorsolateral prefrontal cortex section is powerfully activated in folks that non-public a immoderate degree of strength of will or electricity of mind. This specific same area of the brain is likewise stimulated for the duration of meditation.

Meditation releases the mind's revel in-remarkable hormones, this is great near preventing transient cravings. There are unique chemical materials on the difficulty of endorphins and dopamine in our mind which is probably released on the same time as we get our "immediate fixes." These are the stress-busting chemical substances that motive to fight strain.

When you meditate, you spark off the ones chemical substances and fight pressure without searching out right away gratification or pleasure. Meditation releases the ones chemical substances in a greater healthful and a greater herbal manner, due to this limiting your urges or cravings. This continuously ultimately ultimately ends up growing your electricity of mind and backbone even in addition.

Step 6 - Spend Time With Friends, Family, And Your Pet

Human beings are social creatures. Everything we do is focused in some unspecified time in the future of the fact that we want to connect to every particular. We've built big networks and statistics highways for precisely this purpose. Mindfulness practices assist you understand how interconnected the entirety is.

You will apprehend that the whole thing in this international is created and related to every different. Look at how the surroundings exists. There is a meals chain, and this has a circularity to it, with the animal on top in the long run nourishing the difficulty at the bottom. Life is spherical and the entirety is installed.

As you forge connections with unique people, exercising the 8 pillars of mindfulness. Listen at the side of your entire being in place of definitely looking beforehand to your turn to speak. Nurture and cope with a few shape of life in your private time. What I advise is that even a easy act of being involved for a plant or a domestic dog will deliver more which means that in your life.

Research shows that people want to attend to each unique and need to like and be loved. Older individuals who live in assisted dwelling facilities stay longer after they want to take care of a plant or a puppy. Life in the long run sustains existence.

The maximum critical people to your life are your own family. They want to be on the very top of your precedence list, and that they have got to be the cause you may't wait to get domestic at the give up of the day. When you start getting too busy and you can not find out time to your family, a few element desires to trade. Remind yourself why you visit art work every day. Sure, your profession is essential, however go through in thoughts that every worker in the worldwide can be modified. For your own family, but, you're irreplaceable.

Spending time with buddies, own family or pets permits reduce strain. When you spend time with people you want, you enjoy wonderful approximately yourself.

If you've spent a number of time together collectively collectively with your own family or domestic dog nowadays, you'll locate your self with an extended way a good buy loads a good buy tons less pressure than if you avoided them. You don't need to fear about masses of human beings, however just a few close to ones. You can spend time with as little as one character a day, and I don't care if it's collectively together at the side of your boss, your first rate friend, or possibly your cat, dog, fowl, or goldfish. When you spend time with a person you need, you beautify your degree of happiness and reduces stress.

It is right enough if you don't have any buddies or own family; you can spend time alongside aspect your pup. Being alongside issue your domestic canine is a terrific way to decrease your stress levels. Researchers have showed that 56% of owners see a lower strain diploma after they have offered a puppy. A lot of that is because of the truth whilst you are spherical animals, there may be no pressure on you. You don't need to carry out, and you may sincerely be yourself.

Although you could not have any family or pals to spend time with and you can't come up with the cash for a doggy, you can go out and meet new pals. Though many people also can need to as an possibility stay at home with friends and circle of relatives, it's far essential to socialize and meet new humans. Meeting new human beings encourages you to growth your horizons, and it's far one of the splendid techniques to reduce strain. Make extraordinary you spend time with buddies you acquire as real with, or you can hazard strolling right right proper proper right into a entice.

When you meet a tough and speedy of new human beings, you'll phrase how loads better you sense. Spending time with friends and your doggy will will can help you revel in outstanding about yourself each and every day.Family time is what terrific memories are made from, and also you don't need to be a magnate to expose your family an great time. Here are a few mind for a manner you may de-pressure, spend time collectively together together with your own family, and feature a wonderful work-lifestyles balance:

Go Camping - Nothing beats the outstanding outside, however if you may't get to a campsite, pitch a tent in the outside and characteristic fun sitting below the stars growing a tune songs and eating s'mores.

Play Board Games - Switch off the TV and acquire anybody spherical for a fun board sport night time. This way, you get to interact with, snort with, and function a laugh alongside aspect your circle of relatives in choice to actually sharing the equal vicinity as you do your very personal subjects.

Get Fit - Getting out and transferring is some other superb manner to spend time together. Get everybody within the pool, play volleyball at the seaside, play baseball in the park, or take dance education collectively.

Whatever interest you do together, make certain it's miles interactive and is all about spending satisfactory time collectively. A healthful own family existence is the glue that holds you together while lifestyles gets hard. After all, it's far your circle of relatives who facilitates you unconditionally at the same time as you're forced about paintings or something else. While you have to offer your paintings the time and interest this is due, you must also show your circle of relatives the identical care and interest. By enacting a top notch paintings-balance, you will now not satisfactory be having a laugh, prioritizing what is essential, showing gratitude, and revitalizing your self, but you can moreover be challenge pressure manipulate.

Step 7 - Eat Healthy Food For Your Nerves

Food is such an vital part of our lives, but we cope with it with very little care. The schooling and consumption of food is often handled as a chore and we very rarely reflect onconsideration on meals as gasoline for our our our bodies.

Mindful consuming begins proper from the instant you flow grocery buying. I imply grocery shopping for, as in buying uncooked factors after which cooking them into food, not visiting your nearest rapid-food restaurant or attempting to find a few aspect that can be microwaved into some thing barely suitable for consuming.

Processed meals and chemical components have ruined our palettes to the volume that we do now not even taste actual meals anymore. When you first switch to an entire meals weight loss plan, you'll note which you won't be able to flavor a whole lot of the food you consume. This is because of the truth the flavors decided in processed food are raised to an bad diploma and people food are entire of sugar. The net end end end result is that your flavor buds were dulled and that they want stimulation which will determine out what it's far you're eating.

When purchasing, take it gradual to have a observe the brilliant shades of food available. Marvel at the versions in texture, length and shapes of every component. I'm not advocating changing to veganism or a few factor of the sort. Ultimately, the entirety we eat is food and this includes animals as well. Whether that is best with you or not is up on your ideals. Your motive must be to eat as balanced a diet regime as viable and this indicates which includes meals from fantastic meals groups and mixing as many colours into your food as viable.

This is a neat trick to discern out how balanced your healthy eating plan is surely.

The more severa the feel and colours in your meals, the higher the chances are that you're hitting your dietary goals. Isn't it notable how nature has given us this clean manner of identifying this even as now not having to walk around with a calculator all the time?

As you put together your meals, infuse it with love and desire for it to offer nutrients and lifestyles to absolutely everyone who devour it. When cooking, have a have a look at how the feel of the food adjustments and the manner some of these severa substances come together below warm temperature to shape a unmarried dish. I'm now not seeking to get you to end up a chef proper proper right here, however the way raw elements come together to shape a whole absolutely is a thoughts-blowing technique.

Where is your mind at the same time as you're ingesting your food typically? Probably on the TV or distracted with some thing else. Mealtimes are treated as a chore in most families and this certainly is a shame. Even if the whole circle of relatives comes together for a meal, the motive isn't to experience the food, it's far to talk approximately our day and to settle any lingering troubles.

Take the time to word what your food in reality tastes like and the way it feels in your mouth. Acknowledge that this food is going inner you to gas you and is a key contributor to your health. In current-day-day society, we've a truely terrible relationship with meals. Thanks to the rise of social media, our diets are beneath immoderate scrutiny and masses of meals corporations are demonized.

Some devour only carbs, and some consume fine fats. Some declare juicing is the extremely good and there's a few issue known as the fruit-primarily based definitely food regimen as properly. Understand that each one food is meals. It doesn't bear in mind what you devour so long as it is as in reality sourced as possible and which you consume it inside the right quantities. Even junk food has its area, thinking about the reality that consuming the occasional burger will help you experience better.

Ultimately, that's what meals is meant to do. Make you experience pinnacle approximately dwelling. Seek to acquire a country of stability collectively along side your meals and it's going to go returned the pick out to you thru actual health.

In order to attain pinnacle universal performance to your each day activities, you need to devour healthy.

Food and dietary supplements are effective processes to help prevent and control pressure-associated signs and symptoms. This is due to the truth they are able to trade the way we revel in approximately ourselves, our recognition, relationships and regular outlook on existence.

By ingesting the proper food, we can also help to lessen, or now not much less than, decrease the outcomes of stress in our lives.

What additives are we speakme approximately? Some of the outstanding meals for pressure encompass substances rich in antioxidants—like nuts and fruit. Antioxidants help to neutralize unfastened radicals inside the frame, which guard the frame, and maintain it healthy.

Given that pressure lowers the immune machine and will growth the threat for particular ailments, what may you're saying approximately the efficacy of a plan to address stress, with food? Eating a eating regimen immoderate in antioxidants permits to lessen the awful outcomes of stress.

What meals do this? Foods like nuts and fruit. So, permit's talk approximately nuts— like walnuts and almonds. Walnuts are especially properly- recounted for his or her antioxidant content material fabric. They are excessive in the vital fatty acid amino-acid arginine. This can act as an anticoagulant, decreasing blood stress and enhancing glide. If you are going to select one food to devour, those are the nuts to select. They are also very immoderate in vitamins E, it clearly is a strong antioxidant that is placed in such ingredients as avocados, spinach, broccoli, asparagus, and sunflower seeds.

Free radicals are long-hooked up in our our bodies at the identical time as we're beneath strain. So, if you need to avoid pressure altogether, get enough loose fatty acids (which are observed in food like avocados, walnuts, eggs, salmon, and cod) and fortified factors like breakfast cereals and breads, and reduce the consumption of substances that would be causing you pressure.

Foods like bananas are immoderate in B-vitamins.

These play an essential function in pressure control due to the reality they help the frame better address stress. Vitamin B (at the side of discovered in bananas) decreases the results of pressure with the aid of developing serotonin.

And studies furthermore shows that a food regimen excessive in food plan B lets in to lower the threat for despair.

If you need to keep away from pressure, it's miles essential to consume elements wealthy in nutrition B12, along side salmon, tuna, eggs, and hen.

Some components are wealthy in magnesium include Bananas, chocolate, beans, avocado, and dried fruit, inclusive of raisins and prunes are rich property of magnesium, a temper stabilizer that is exceedingly powerful in the fight in opposition to pain and strain. Dried fruits are loaded with potassium, that could be a herbal diuretic and muscle relaxer.

So why is magnesium so important? Magnesium permits to loosen up blood vessels, which lets in to save you a flare-up of the pressure reaction, in addition to helps balance the body's response to stress.

The key to decreasing the outcomes of strain is to have wholesome and regular levels of those vitamins that assist lessen stress.

Chapter 4: Additional Ways To Reduce Your Stress For The Long Term

Step eight - Reduce Caffeine Intake

Caffeine promotes the production of adrenaline that, in some unspecified time in the future of intervals of strain, is a supply of "fight or flight," the reaction mechanism that makes us each combat, flight or freeze. It is beneficial to slight caffeine intake determined in cola, red bull, and espresso or tea. The every day recommendation is to eat at maximum four hundred mg of caffeine, equal to about four cups of espresso in step with day.

Caffeine changed into diagnosed to provide skin extra buzz for its antioxidant pastime and wonderful ability to neutralize unfastened radicals. It additionally permits inhibit the pimples breakout enzyme. In addition, caffeine is likewise an anti-inflammatory agent used to address different pores and skin irritations.

Caffeine can intensify emotions of anxiety due to the fact it is a stimulant, so every time you enjoy the need to loosen up, update that glass of caffeine with a cup of something soothing. Chamomile and peppermint have soothing houses that reduce anxiety and sell rest, and loads of people use them to help themselves go to sleep at night time. You can use those herbs proactively by means of using developing a cup of chamomile or peppermint tea a ordinary a part of your day. The subsequent time you're feeling careworn, take ten mins to boil water, brew, and sip your creation.

If you need to unfastened yourself from being absolutely inspired by way of demanding conditions, it's far super to lessen your intake of caffeine.

Here's the way it works: If your combat-or-flight response is heightened, your pressure stages may be excessive. Caffeine will make you sense more confused, most vital to intake of more caffeine in order to help you experience less compelled. This can bring about a downward spiral of dependency and craving.

There is likewise a non-clinical manner to explain this: Caffeine (and coffee, for that do not forget) consists of a mildly radioactive detail referred to as "cobalt-60." This substance is a byproduct of nuclear reactors. Whenever we devour it in espresso or tea or soda, the radioactive cobalt-60 seeps into our DNA, converting our genes. Now, we aren't talking about most important structural alternate in our DNA in this example, however diffused, minor adjustments that could growth our vulnerability to stress. We additionally understand that the extra pressure we're under, the more prone we are to ailments and degenerative illnesses. All of that is due to the cobalt-60, which we consume with our day by day cup of coffee.

What we are able to do, then, to interrupt the downward spiral of dependency and yearning is to reduce our caffeine intake or perhaps stop. The greater stress we revel in, the more prone we're to sickness, and the extra we're able to crave our caffeine recuperation. We desire that thru lowering down on caffeine or quitting it, our strain tiers will circulate down so we are able to restore our genes to their unique nation.

Other than caffeine, there are liquids you may take to help you lessen your pressure. Yes, liquids. Read on and discover more.

I'm going to list some. You may likely find out a number of those tastier, and it'll in all likelihood assist you lighten up more as nicely. These are:

Jasmine Green Tea: This is one of the most thrilling beverages close to anxiety and pressure. It's a warmness and soothing aroma of jasmine flower which will will permit you to loosen up after a tiring day.

Lavender: Really stressing? Just boil this aromatic herb after which sip it at the element of water. This will allow you to understand the wonders of lavender, and will make your day greater bearable for you.

Lemon: Lemon is a completely not unusual drink in phrases of lowering stress. This is a fresh, mind-bending and a totally wonderful enjoy for you. If you are forced, drink some lemon water and you'll definitely enjoy it.

Red wine: Red wine has pretty some iron and is frequently fermented. This offers you lots of energy, and even as you are eating it, it's also going to lessen your stress. So, next time you're forced out, drink some red wine. You can not pass wrong.

Green tea: Green tea end up presented #1 in a list of food that help reduce stress. So, next time you are burdened out, it's miles important to strive it.

Vodka and Orange Juice: Do you need vodka? Orange juice? You may additionally count on orange juice would not go along with vodka. But, it's miles a chemical reaction. It's real that in case you combination orange juice with vodka it's going to reduce your strain.

Ginger: If you want to drink ginger tea, you want to genuinely remember eating ginger pix. It's exceptional.

Red grape juice: Yes, you heard me right. Red grape juice will lessen your stress and it'll also make you experience active. So, in case you're burdened out, brew red grape juice, and lap it up!

Banana: The banana is the ideal fruit for a builder's healthy dietweight-reduction plan, or furthermore for a runner's healthy eating plan. Healers, which may be normally known as shamans in the beyond, used to devour bananas, for the motive that they want to accumulate their energy after an entire day of healing. And, it labored. It gave them plenty of electricity. Besides, you may make a banana shake if you really need to reduce your pressure. Bananas are also a supply of iron and will consequently offer you with loads of strength.

Water: Yes, a tumbler of water will do.

Bottom line is that there are numerous one-of-a-kind liquids you could take that will help you reduce your strain. You'll should strive out certainly one of a kind kinds of drinks to discover which one will lessen your stress inside the pleasant manner and make you enjoy higher.

Chapter 5: Listen To Soothing Music

How does it take region that music influences us and our brains?

Music has an impact on humans due to the fact it's far an opportunity to language. Music has consistent patterns, and that is why even as we be aware of rhythmic music our tendency is to transport in stay overall performance with it.

Music additionally operates on our emotions and connects to our emotions. Music links up with areas of our mind, which then translates into sensations. The scale of feeling is massive, beginning from extremely good pride to crying.

It is famous that pregnant women regularly play tune for the fetus inner their womb. The music offers the female sensations that secrete hormones that acquire the fetus, growing a connection most of the sounds and the sensations.

Musical scale additionally has significance. Music in a minor scale will usually make us experience nostalgic or wake up recollections of a unhappy event we skilled, rather than music in a joyous maximum crucial scale.

Let's pass lower again to the "Koolulam" task. Out of instructional hobby, I signed up for one in every in their instructions. I felt incredible pleasure. When all those people sang, I had a sense of friendship and togetherness. This is also natural. Shared creating a song motives individuals to release hormones, specially oxytocin, which causes a feeling of elation.

It is much like the feeling you may revel in if you attend a agency in an African-American church. Their developing a tune is a exciting experience that could cause a country of meditation.

Curiously, it doesn't rely if the track is sorrowful or joyous, the important element is that after the choir sings all collectively the sounds contact us and launch the "correct feeling" hormones.

You do not need to understand the tune, sincerely experience it. Listening to track may be a massive device for lowering pressure, in particular if we integrate it with one of the exclusive techniques stated in the e-book.

Try making your playlists on the give up of the day and play song you like. Another preference is attending public growing a music activities, mass growing a song inclusive of a "Koolulam" occasion, or specific social group creating a track.

Music can soothe us, excite us, and make us experience extra comfortable, however it may moreover offend us in notable techniques. The melody and rhythm permit the thoughts to be calmed, relaxed, and placed the thoughts proper right into a high-quality u . S . Of being. Music has the ability to react at the frame thru modifications in coronary heart fee, blood pressure, respiratory or even blood flow. Changes in respiratory and coronary coronary heart charge monitor the results of tune on arousal main to the notion that music may be used as a device to reduce pressure. The tune need to actually have a splendid rhythm to it. Meditation song, for instance, can be very calming and soothing to someone anywhere that man or woman is.

Stress is due to different factors like circle of relatives, friends, paintings and really many extra factors. It takes a toll at the mind, body, and soul while collected and even as it hits difficult. It can reason lifelong health troubles and it have to be researched and brought into consideration with caution. Listening to song will have every wonderful and horrible results. It can sooth a person who's compelled or it could initiate more strain based without a doubt on the song. It can be a topic of conflict of phrases at home, inside the administrative center, on the barber save, within the car and everywhere else. The results of strain produced by way of the usage of song can be reduced by way of way of the usage of it efficiently steady with some researchers that I will talk about in a chunk.

Music can be used creatively for the coolest of the human beings on this worldwide because of the fact it may be used as a deliver of rest and discount of pressure. Some studies have validated that paying attention to tune can be used for restoration functions for ailments like despair. One of the most reliable music clinical medical doctors inside the global, Gabriel Fiorentino, modified into able to create a song remedy software application with the help of neuroscience and psychology. Mary Ziegler is a pioneer in developing a very particular form of tune treatment that is the usage of tune. The use of track allows to stimulate the mind and stimulate the brain to reap the great diploma of thinking. Music may be used to stimulate key factors of the mind which can be the visible mind, cognitive thoughts, auditory mind, and motor brain. These mind areas are responsible for making plans, thinking, and unique crucial talents.

Technology has enabled technological comprehend-the way to discover the power of song. The use of music remedy has been used to help analyzing, manage, auditory processing, cognitive development, and speech. Music has been used to enhance results or maybe to cope with sicknesses of the mind which incorporates Alzheimer's disorder, Tourette's syndrome, epilepsy, schizophrenia, and autistic spectrum problems. Music can also also be used to reduce pain and the pain that is due to the shortage of nerve cells in the spinal cord. Music additionally may be used to help recover from Alzheimer's disorder sufferers.

Music can dramatically have an effect on the body thru many terrific associated mechanisms. The mind is a splendid a part of the dwelling body and it's miles chargeable for many vital skills which incorporates memory, idea, coordination, and plenty greater. The autonomic apprehensive device controls absolutely considered one of a type internal body structures that want to be functioning if you need to feature. Changes in the hormonal, immune, and cardiovascular structures can be suffering from track. Heart price, blood stress, and respiratory fee may be all altered through the use of music. When a person listens to tune the body can block ache indicators and blood float to the muscle tissues.

Music has been applied in healing for heaps of years typically for non secular or non secular motives. It has excellent effects on people because of the manner they interpret the tune. The thoughts is constantly inspired by means of the tune produced and it permits in calming you down, specially even as pressured.

Step 10 - Get More Sleep

Good outstanding sleep is important to normal every day functioning. It is likewise advocated to workout meditation about 1/2 an hour earlier than mattress, the use of considered one in every of your preferred strategies.

Strange as it could sound, sleep is a high-quality device for handling pressure. When we are confused, we are in a vicious negative cycle. When we are very disturbed (particularly even as pressure is chronic), our mind also intrude into our minds at night time time and we will find out it hard to go to sleep. Due to a loss of sleep we become extra worn-out and the gathered fatigue makes it hard for us to control well with pressure and its recurrence.

Quality sleep is crucial for smooth the thoughts. Do no longer fall asleep with the tv blaring inside the ancient beyond, and do no longer have a mobile phone close by. Sleep brilliant can be improved first and vital thru manner of getting cushty sleeping situations, a right pillow, blanket, suitable low lighting fixtures, and silence round you.

The advice that is repeated in almost all studies inside the field is to fall asleep at a normal time for a complete eight hours a night time. A nap in the afternoon, the "powernap" is likewise essential.

The powernap is brief-time period day time sleep (in preference to in the night hours) of about twenty minutes on common. Longer durations will result in the sleep onset nation (R.E.M.) that isn't always suitable during day time.

Studies have shown that personnel who take a powernap at a few stage in the day show first-rate development in productiveness. The development is apparent in factors including creativity, seen notion, data processing, and associative thinking. Such sleep moreover improves alertness.

I in particular propose the powernap for folks who are very busy in some unspecified time in the future of the day and want more power to get through the day.

There are countries wherein that is an established manner of life: In Spain it's far the Siesta, in Italy the Riposo, and within the United States, corporations that supply time and idea to enhancing the first-class of the lives of their worker, have installation areas positive for powernaps and meditation.

But there's a easy approach to avoid a vicious cycle: the capability to get sufficient sleep. The body produces sufficient cortisol, the stress hormone. When our frame falls asleep, the overall level of strain hormones decreases, which in flip decreases strain in us. Therefore, sufficient sleep reduces stress and permits us get over the each day burdens we stock. The loss of sleep is a notable reason of stress in itself, and moreover one of the elements for terrific highbrow, emotional and physical ailments.

And subsequently, the terrible trouble approximately pressure is that it regularly takes location at night. In order to get some peace of mind via falling asleep, you need to wait till the next day. Therefore, we want to learn how to go to sleep quicker (explanation underneath).

Try to installation a everyday ritual – your private sleeping ritual. To get organized for sleep, do the following:

1. Place your tongue at the top palate, simply in the lower back of the the front

teeth. – Try to move away it there at some point of the whole habitual.

2. Breathe out out of your mouth – one very lengthy exhale. 1. Keep your mouth closed and inhale through your nose for 4 or five seconds to take greater oxygen into the frame.

2. Hold your breath for seven seconds to allow oxygen to penetrate the bloodstream.

3. Open your mouth and exhale for eight or ten seconds to slow your coronary heart fee and launch greater carbon dioxide from your lungs.

4. Repeat this several instances and maximum likely you may awaken refreshed within the morning.

Practice:

1. Seating – If there's no snug bed or sofa available, you could doze off seated in a cushty armchair. Your legs need to be multiplied, and it is exceptional to apply a cushty pillow for your returned and head

that may be saved inside the workplace for this motive.

2.   Turn off telephones and computer systems – Earplugs will help muffle sound. Darken the room, but no longer virtually. If it's miles tough to make the room darkish, you could use a watch mask product of healthy material. If you are not an earplug enthusiast, there are terrific headphones that isolate external noises.

3.   Quiet time – Some human beings opt for whole silence, however others select "white noise." Specific sound frequency may be decided on with committed apps (down load a "white noise" app out of your iPhone or Android cellphone).

4.   Temperature – Studies have verified that the top of the street temperature for sleep is a fab sixty- to sixty-six degrees Fahrenheit or seventeen to nineteen degrees Celsius, so it's miles truely beneficial to cover your self with a moderate blanket.

five. Routine – Set a regular time for this moderate sleep in the route of the day. It is specially applicable to have it after lunch, but be careful not to devour caffeine, sugar, fats-saturated factors, or sugary drinks at the least an hour in advance than the nap.

6. Apps – There are quite a few apps that help with sleep: SLEEPSMART, a nice, free app that has alternatives for playing a "white noise" sound, putting an alarm, in addition to Relax Melodies. Google has a significant desire to test out.

Chapter 6: How Stress Takes a Toll at the Brain and Behavior?

Stress affects your mind inside the following techniques:

Brain Structure: Experiments furthermore mounted that lengthy-term changes within the structure and function of the mind might also need to end result from persistent strain. The thoughts's gray rely, it is responsible for better-order thinking inclusive of desire-making and hassle-fixing, is made from neurons and assist cells. However, the mind additionally includes "white depend," it truly is manufactured from all the axons that communicate facts with other factors of the mind. The fatty, white layer known as myelin that envelopes the axons that boost up the electric alerts had to switch statistics at some point of the brain offers white rely its name. The overproduction of myelin determined by means of way of the researchers inside the presence of persistent stress does no longer absolutely motive a brief-term shift inside the balance among white and grey remember; it could moreover purpose long-time period structural abnormalities in the thoughts.

The researcher on the back of these trials, Psychologist Daniela Kaufer, believes that based completely at the patterning of white depend you get early in existence, you are building a mind this is each resilient or very touchy to intellectual troubles.

Brain Shrinkage: Stress can purpose shrinkage in elements of the mind related to emotion regulation, metabolism, and memory, even in in any other case wholesome humans. While many people associate bad consequences with unexpected, excessive pressure because of lifestyles-converting sports (which consist of a car twist of destiny, natural catastrophe, or the dearth of existence of a loved one), researchers don't forget that ordinary pressure, which clearly all of us seem to face, can contribute to numerous intellectual issues over the years.

Researchers from Yale University studied one hundred healthy individuals who shared facts on worrying opinions of their existence in a unmarried have a look at. The researchers determined that strain caused much less gray depend in the prefrontal cortex, a mind vicinity related to willpower and emotions.

Chronic, normal pressure seems to have little impact on thoughts amount on its very very own, however it seems to render human beings more sensitive to mind shrinkage while confronted with immoderate, catastrophic stresses.

Distinct kinds of stress have precise results at the thoughts. Emotional attention is suffering from cutting-edge worrying recollections (activity loss, automobile injuries). Mood facilities are greater suffering from worrying opinions (loss of life of a cherished one, massive illness).

Killing Brain Cells: Researchers have positioned that a single socially annoying occasion can motive new neurons to die in the hippocampus of the mind. The hippocampus is a mind place that is strongly related to emotion, reminiscence, and getting to know. It is likewise taken into consideration certainly one of regions of the mind wherein neurogenesis, or the development of new thoughts cells, occurs all the time.

The researchers experimented with the aid of manner of setting greater youthful rats in a cage with character rats for 20 mins. The child rat turned into in the end subjected to aggressiveness from the cage's greater professional people. The cortisol tiers of the more youthful rats had been found to be up to six instances greater than the ones of rats who had no longer long gone through a stressful social stumble upon.

Further research positioned that, at the same time as younger rats exposed to stress created the same amount of latest neurons as those who had now not been uncovered to strain, the type of nerve cells emerge as appreciably decreased according to week later. Stress does now not appear to affect the producing of new neurons, however it does have an effect on the survival of those cells.

Depression: Chronic, or extended-time period, stress may be horrible on its very very own, but it can additionally reason melancholy, a temper situation that reasons you to feel gloomy and tired of sports which you commonly experience. Depression may also want to have an effect on your urge for meals, sleep patterns, and capacity to consciousness. A giant stressor, at the aspect of a divorce event a exceptional financial shift, is a high-quality stressor that throws the psyche off balance. According to a researcher, in case you maintain growing your stress tiers, some aspect will occur, and the most not unusual very last results is depression.

Anxiety: Corticotropin and cortisol hormones may also additionally growth anxiety and make contributions to temper problems if strain degrees do no longer lower. Researchers laced the mice's consuming water with corticosterone in a have a look at. They had been able to avoid stressing the mice with the aid of manner of no longer injecting them. The laced water changed into given to 3 mice for 17 or 18 days, simulating extended-term stress hormone exposure. The different mice, however, best obtained the boosted water for in the end. The mice were given assessments and not the use of a education to prepare them for them. Mice in a dark region of a cage have been given the possibility to discover a sparkly, open a part of the cage in a single test. The mice who fed on the tainted water on a every day foundation have been more careful about coming into the open location. The reluctance have turn out to be seemed as nervousness with the resource of the researchers.

If you have had pressure for a while, you may relate to at the least some of the above issues. Now let's try and understand the anger.

2.2 Inside Anger

Anger manifests in our our our bodies further to our mind, just like special emotions. When we feel furious, our our our bodies undergo a complicated set of physiological (frame) sports.

Emotions begin in our brains' amygdala, this is almond-usual systems. The amygdala is the part of the mind that detects risks to our properly-being and issues an alarm while risks are detected, prompting us to take protecting measures. The amygdala is so exceptional at warning us approximately risks that it gets us reacting in advance than the cortex (the part of the thoughts that deals with mind and judgment) can verify if our response is wise. In specific phrases, our brains are constructed to compel us to act in advance than we can honestly apprehend the ramifications of our moves. This is not a justification for terrible conduct; human beings can and do manage their aggressive inclinations, and with exercising, you could as properly. Instead, it indicates that effectively managing anger is a taught capacity in desire to a few component we are born with.

Your frame's muscle organizations hectic up as you grow to be enraged. Catecholamines, which is probably neurotransmitter chemical substances, are produced on your mind, producing a burst of electricity that may final for numerous minutes. The regular outraged impulse to take brief protective movement is the give up result of this burst of electricity. Your coronary coronary heart charge, blood strain, and respiratory price all increase on the same 2nd. Increased blood go with the float for your limbs and extremities prepares you for bodily interest, which can also moreover motive your face to flush. Your reputation narrows to the deliver of your rage. Nothing else may be able to maintain your interest for prolonged. Additional mind neurotransmitters and hormones (inclusive of adrenaline and noradrenaline) are released in fast succession, resulting in an arousal nation that lasts for a long term. You are organized to fight now.

Although your emotions can spiral out of manipulate, your prefrontal cortex, that is positioned right now underneath your forehead, can preserve them in test. The prefrontal cortex is in fee of judgment if the amygdala is in price of emotion. Emotions may be grew to emerge as off thru the left prefrontal cortex. It acts as a manager, making sure that the whole lot is in order. Learning the way to help your prefrontal cortex take manage of your amygdala so that you can control the manner you react to anger emotions is step one in gaining control over your anger.

Now permit's dive into the motives why you need to hire your left prefrontal cortex.

Effects of Anger

Anger is a powerful emotion that has behavioral manifestations. It may be a essential tool for survival, but it can moreover motive huge issues in the long run thru knocking the mind's associated with thinking, feeling, conduct, and relationships. It is a forceful, uncomfortable, and awkward reaction to what you bear in mind you studied is a provocation, harm, or chance. When non-public obstacles are violated, anger is prompted. Anger is, thru the usage of nature, a caution signal to guard oneself from fear, disappointment, or suffering, both cognitively, behaviorally, or physically, from an externally risky publicity thru movement decided on of one's private volition. Anger could have most important effects on your life and behavior. Let's talk them:

- How Anger takes a Toll on the Body?

Your body is at danger because of anger within the following techniques:

Heart Problems: Most unstable effect of anger is in your coronary coronary coronary heart fitness. According to a scientific psychiatry instructor, the hazard of struggling a coronary heart attack doubles within the hours following an indignant outburst. Moreover, it's far researched that coronary coronary heart infection is connected to repressed anger at the same time as you specific it indirectly or visit exquisite lengths to manipulate it. According to 1 check, the ones who have anger proneness as a character function have two times the threat of cardiovascular sickness as their less angry opposite numbers.

Immune System: If you are mad all of the time, you certainly may find your self feeling sick more regularly. In one take a look at, Harvard University scientists determined that during wholesome human beings, virtually recalling an irritated revel in from their past introduced about a six-hour dip in ranges of the antibody immunoglobulin A, the cells' first line of protection toward contamination. Moreover, in keeping with an Ohio State University observe, folks that had a great deal less manipulate over their anger healed wounds more slowly. Researchers gave blisters to 98 humans and observed that individuals who had less manipulate over their anger, healed slower after eight days. Furthermore, at a few stage within the blistering operation, the ones subjects had higher levels of cortisol (a pressure hormone), implying that they have been additionally greater agitated through demanding sports.

Respiratory System: Even if you do no longer smoke, being a continually irritated and antagonistic person would probable harm your lungs. Using a hostility scale scoring approach to quantify anger levels and observe any changes within the men's lung feature, a set of Harvard University scientists studied 670 guys for 8 years. The person men who rated themselves due to the fact the maximum hostile had hundreds decrease lung capacity, growing their threat of respiration troubles. Stress hormones, which can be related to emotions of anger, are notion to reason irritation within the airways, steady with the check.

Life Expectancy: A 17-one year study with the useful resource of the University of Michigan positioned that couples who maintain their anger in had decrease existence length than those who particular their anger brazenly. According to a observe, strain is inextricably associated with general health. You will stay a shorter existence if you are demanding and livid.

- How Anger takes a Toll on the Brain and Behavior?

Anger influences your thoughts within the following techniques:

Anxiety: If you're a worrier, you need to be conscious that fear and anger can coexist. Anger can growth symptoms of a generalized tension disorder (GAD), a state of affairs defined with the useful resource of manner of immoderate and uncontrollable worry that interferes with a person's normal existence, in keeping with a 2012 test published inside the magazine Cognitive Behavior Therapy. Not simplest did sufferers with GAD have better levels of anger, but hostility — specifically internalized, unexpressed anger — have become connected to the severity of GAD signs and symptoms.

Depression: Depression has been associated in severa studies to aggression and furious outbursts, specially in men. Passive rage is regular in despair, in that you ruminate over some issue however in no manner do some thing high quality approximately it. Anger issues in spouses and wives were explored in a unmarried observe from the University of Washington: School of Nursing. Previous studies has connected anger issues and depressive signs and symptoms to all primary motives of mortality, consistent with the researchers. Women, however, had a stronger link amongst anger and depressive signs, while guys had a stronger link amongst anger and fitness problems.

Social Depravity: Being angry all of the time has most essential social and emotional prices further to physical health implications. People who are hostile and irritated are a good deal a whole lot much less in all likelihood to have real supportive relationships than folks that are a good buy a great deal much less poor. Most importantly, chronic anger inhibits closeness in personal relationships and special own family contributors are greater guarded and much plenty less able to loosen up in ugly conditions.

While this could not appear to be a horrific destiny to have, keep in thoughts that studies continuously demonstrates that having healthy supportive relationships with circle of relatives, pals, coworkers, and associates is important for suitable fitness. Having the social aid of one's peers might in all likelihood help one keep away from intellectual problems as well as large fitness issues like coronary heart illness. When people have vast social manual, they're a good buy much less likely to be stricken by the use of debilitating despair.

The physiological reaction to anger and arousal advanced to assist people in handling bodily risks. Physical aggression, but, isn't typically a appropriate response in cutting-edge way of existence. This is in particular right in the extra public elements of your lifestyles, together with your encounters at art work. You will nearly genuinely be fired if you verbally attack your manager. Similarly, if you get out of your car and attack a purpose force who has reduce you off, you can emerge as in court docket. Uncontrollable rage can motive interest loss, circle of relatives separation, or even jail. Individuals who are not capable of manipulate their disruptive, violent conduct are more likely to face now not simplest extra fitness dangers but furthermore maximum essential social problems.

I need to quit this chapter at the be conscious that stress and anger can break your bodily and intellectual health. The subsequent two chapters will help you do away with this gradual existence-threatening poison out of your lifestyles.

Chapter 7: Managing an Angry Brain

Managing your anger does now not exempt you from being indignant. Rather, it includes reading to recognize, control, and express anger in a healthful and excellent way. Anger manage is a capability that may be determined with the useful resource of anybody. There is commonly place for improvement, even if you expect you have got have been given your anger under control.

Let's debunk some myths about anger in advance than we bypass ahead:

- Anger Is a Bad Feeling

All of the primary feelings are important and hardwired into our brains. Stuffing them isn't always a top notch concept. One way the frame communicates its necessities is through emotion. However, this doesn't advise that we need to automatically react. We can reply greater successfully and flip topics spherical if we take a look at the sensation.

- It is Okay to Blow Up

When we're angry, our minds can also moreover additionally rationalize something. When your mind is hijacked through anger, it is hard to cope with problems. You can rationalize your angry outbursts by means of using telling your self, "She made me angry." It's no longer actual, and it does now not assist subjects.

- Anger is all in your head.

Anger is greater than simplest a intellectual u . S .. Consider the final time you have been definitely enraged. Your heart charge probable raised, your face flushed, and your fingers shook. This is due to the reality anger triggers a physiological reaction, which in flip fuels angry mind and aggressive moves. To reduce competitive outbursts, you need to discover ways to calm your frame—and your thoughts.

- Ignoring your anger will make it disappear.

Anger suppression is not appropriate, both. Smiling to mask your dissatisfaction, rejecting your furious sentiments, or allowing others to deal with you badly to preserve the peace can also moreover purpose your anger to spiral inward. In addition, suppressed rage has been linked to a number of physical and intellectual health issues, together with excessive blood stress and despair.

- Some people are simply born with a awful mood that they cannot manage.

Angry emotions are the result of tales which can be regularly overlooked or forgotten and don't have something to do with the "motives" we tell ourselves for being irritated.

You may also moreover additionally keep in mind that expressing your rage is healthful, that the ones spherical you are overly sensitive, that your anger is justifiable, or which you need to expose your anger to advantage recognize. However, rage is more likely to have a terrible impact on how others see you, impair your judgment, and hinder your achievement.

So allow's examine the keys to tame your anger.

three.1 Are You Ready for a Change?

Choosing to take manage of your anger in area of allowing it to control you necessitates a radical exam of ways you have were given been reacting whilst you are angry. Do you will be willing to scream and yell or to mention nasty, suggest, and disrespectful topics? Do you hurl devices, kick or punch walls, or damage things? Do you need to hit someone, injure your self, or push and shove wonderful human beings around?

Most human beings who've troubles controlling their temper do not need to react on this way. They are embarrassed with the aid of way of their movements and consider that it does now not mirror their actual self, their tremendous selves.

Everyone has the capability to alternate, however simplest once they want to. Consider what you may benefit in case you make a massive shift within the way you deal with your anger. Is it viable to have extra self-recognize? Is it possible to benefit extra recognize from others? Spending plenty a lot much less time indignant and pissed off? A more laid-decrease again mindset in the direction of lifestyles? It can assist in remembering why you need to make the exchange.

It is also a exceptional concept to remind you that exchange takes time, try, and staying power. It is not going to reveal up . Managing anger calls for the improvement of latest talents and responses. It enables to exercise again and again over again with any competencies, consisting of mastering the piano or gambling basketball.

three.2 Exploring Yourself

Identifying the real deliver of your inflammation will will will let you properly supply an reason of your anger, take nice motion, and paintings closer to a solution.

• Is your anger concealing specific emotions like humiliation, uncertainty, shame, harm, or vulnerability?

If you discover yourself reacting with anger in quite some conditions, it is probably that your fury is overlaying your actual emotions. This is especially real in case you grew up in a circle of relatives wherein expressing feelings became frowned upon. You may moreover locate it difficult to widely known emotions aside from anger as an person.

• Anger additionally may be a symptom of anxiety.

Your body engages the "combat or flight" reaction whilst you apprehend a hazard, actual or imagined. The "fight" reaction is regularly manifested as rage or hostility inside the case of the "fight" response. To regulate your reaction, you have to first choose out the supply of your anxiety or fear.

- What you discovered as a infant can be the supply of your anger troubles.

You may also moreover want to assume this is how anger is meant to be expressed in case you see others to your circle of relatives yell, strike every exclusive, or throw objects.

- Anger can be a symptom of a few underlying health issues.

It may be depression, trauma, or chronic pressure (mainly in guys).

There is extra to your anger than meets the attention, consistent with those signs and symptoms:

1. You see opposing viewpoints as a personal project: Do you think your manner is usually accurate and emerge as enraged at the same time as others disagree? If you have got a sturdy need to be in rate or a susceptible ego, you can misread specific viewpoints as a chance in your authority instead of really a selected mindset.

2. You can also have a hard time making compromises: Is it tough a terrific manner to recognize exceptional humans's viewpoints or maybe greater tough that lets in you to concede a issue? If you grew up in a own family wherein anger come to be out of manipulate, you'll likely preserve in mind how the person that modified into the most enraged had been given their way via the use of being the loudest and demanding. Compromise can reason frightening feelings of failure and vulnerability.

three. You find it tough to speak emotions other than anger: Do you are taking delight in being hard and in command? Do you consider you studied you are proof towards feelings like worry, remorse, or disgrace? Everyone has those emotions, so you is probably protective them with rage. It is vital to reconnecting together with your feelings in case you are uncomfortable with severa feelings, disengaged, or stuck on an irritated one-note reaction to subjects.

3.3 Identifying Triggers

While worrying activities do no longer justify anger, spotting how they effect you can assist you are taking manage of your environment and keep away from unneeded annoyance. Examine your every day everyday to peer if there are any sports activities, human beings, and times of day, locations, or conditions that make you angry or livid.

Maybe every time you go out for beverages with a high-quality set of pals, you get right right into a fight. Alternatively, probably the website on line traffic to your each day travel drives you insane. You should likely decide to reorganize your day an excellent manner to higher manage your pressure. Alternatively, you may possibly exercise anger manage strategies in advance than encountering situations which you commonly find out worrying. Doing the ones sports activities sports allow you to amplify your fuse, because of this you may not be caused via a unmarried stressful revel in.

You may also trust that your anger is due to outside assets together with exclusive humans's callous actions or aggravating situations. However, anger problems have plenty much less to do with what takes place to you and extra to do with the manner you interpret and don't forget it.

The following are a few common terrible concept techniques that motive and gasoline anger:

1. Overgeneralizing: It can appear to be this:

"You 'always' interrupt me."

"You 'in no manner' recall what I need."

"'Everyone' seems down on me."

"I am 'in no way' given the credit score I am due."

2. Obsessing over the phrases "need to" and "need to:" Having a inflexible photograph of the way a state of affairs have to or need to spread and being

enraged at the same time as truth fails to wholesome this perfect.

3. Jumping to conclusions and interpreting people's minds: Assuming you "understand" what a person else is questioning or feeling and that they have executed so on cause to upset you, forget approximately your requests, or insult you.

4. Collecting Straws: Looking for topics to be indignant about on the same time as ignoring or brushing apart something beneficial. Allowing tiny irritations to accumulate till you obtain the "very last straw" and explode, normally over some thing insignificant.

five. Blaming: It is constantly someone else's fault whilst some issue unpleasant takes location or is going incorrect. Instead of taking responsibility to your personal lifestyles, you inform yourself, "Life isn't honest," or blame others in your problems.

You might also moreover discover ways to reframe the way you do not forget topics while you discover the highbrow styles that feed your anger. Consider this: What evidence do you have got that the belief is accurate? Is it possible that this isn't the case? Is there a extra effective, realistic mindset on a state of affairs? What might I say to a pal who had the ones thoughts?

3.Four Being Aware of Anger Warning Signs

While it could appear which you become enraged without warning, your frame does show off physical warning signs and signs. You may additionally additionally take efforts to adjust your anger earlier than it spirals out of manage in case you turn out to be privy to your very very personal personal symptoms that your mood is beginning to boil. Pay interest to how your anger makes your frame sense:

- Clenching your jaw or arms
- Knots in your belly
- Feeling flushed or clammy
- Breathing faster

- Pacing or sense the want to stroll spherical
- Headaches
- Having hassle concentrating
- "Seeing red"
- Tensing your shoulders
- Pounding coronary heart

three.Five Learning to Calm Yourself

You can address your anger earlier than it receives out of manage if you recognize the manner to identify the caution indicators that your mood is growing and expect your triggers. There are an entire lot of techniques that may help you in calming down and controlling your anger.

- Concentrate on the bodily manifestations of anger. While it could appear paradoxical, taking note of how your body feels whilst you are furious might likely assist you manage your anger's emotional depth.

• Learn to step away. Trying to win an difficulty or sticking it out in a awful scenario will definitely make you greater enraged. When your anger is increasing, one of the greatest topics you could do is to get out of the situation as rapid as viable.

• Take a damage whilst a dialogue becomes heated. If you enjoy like you're approximately to blow up, you should depart the meeting. If your kids are bothering you, bypass for a stroll. A time-out might be useful in calming your mind and frame.

If you frequently have heated arguments with a person, which includes a friend or member of the family, communicate to them about the want of taking a destroy and restarting whilst you every are feeling calm.

When you need to take a break, offer an reason for which you aren't seeking to keep away from unsightly topics; as a substitute, you're walking on anger manage. When you're disillusioned, it isn't always viable to have a meaningful communicate or remedy a conflict of terms. When you feel greater comfortable, you can keep the communication or cope with the problem.

Setting a completely particular time and location to speak about the situation once more can every so often be beneficial. This gives your colleague, buddy, or member of the family the assurance that the problem may be addressed—just at a later time.

- You can use plenty of relaxation sports activities sports that will help you control your anger. You ought to exercising which one works extremely good for you. Two prominent strategies for lowering anxiety are breathing carrying sports and innovative muscle relaxation.

The fantastic difficulty is that each wearing sports may be finished in a quick quantity of time and with minimum attempt. So, whether or not you're dissatisfied at art work or angry approximately a dinner reservation, you could swiftly and with out hassle allow cross of stress.

It is critical to maintain in thoughts, too, that rest strategies take time to grasp. You might not suppose that they're effective within the starting, or you could surprise if they may be going to be surely right for you. They can, but, turn out to be your pass-to techniques for anger manage with exercise.

- You get a burst of power while you are irritated. Engaging in bodily interest is one of the exquisite methods to place that surge to suitable use. Working out, whether or not or no longer it is a brisk walk or a adventure to the gym allow you to relieve pressure. Regular workout moreover aids in the decompression method. Aerobic pastime reduces anxiety, which may also assist you cope higher with frustration. Exercising additionally assists you to de-muddle your mind. You may also moreover discover that once a long time or a strenuous exercise, you have got a better information of what's bothering you.

- Make use of your senses. To suddenly reduce pressure and take a seat down backtrack, interact your senses of scent, sight, being attentive to, taste, and phone. Looking at a favorite image, relishing a cup of tea, or touching a doggy are all perfect options.

- Humor and playfulness may additionally help you lighten the temper, smooth over disagreements, reframe issues, and hold subjects in attitude at the same time as subjects get irritating. When you are feeling angry in a situation, strive a bit lighthearted comedy. It assist you to speak your message without elevating the alternative individual's safety or hurting their emotions.

It is important, however, which you snigger with the alternative man or woman as opposed to at them. Avoid sarcasm and derogatory humor. If you're uncertain, begin with self-deprecating humor. We all understand individuals who can lightly mock their very own shortcomings. After all, we're all fallible, and we're all liable to making mistakes. So, alternatively of getting furious or growing a fight because of the fact you made a mistake at art work or spilled coffee for the duration of your self, strive developing a funny tale about it. The best character you chance insulting is yourself if the shaggy canine story falls flat or is introduced incorrectly. A potential confrontation might also even emerge as a risk for higher connection and intimacy whilst humor and play are used to alleviate tension and hostility. Sarcasm, however, have to be prevented because of the fact it would harm feelings and make topics worse.

- Manage your thoughts. Your anger is fueled through way of using angry thoughts. "I can not stand it," you will likely think. "This site visitors put off goes to damage everything," you will assume to yourself. Reframe your thoughts even as you find your self considering matters that make you angry. Instead, go through in thoughts the facts and provide some aspect like, "Every day, loads of thousands of motors are on the street." There is probably web page web page visitors jams once in a while." Staying calmer may be as easy as focusing at the records with out throwing in terrible prophecies or twisted exaggerations. You may additionally additionally offer you with a mantra that you can repeat to drown out the thoughts which may be fueling your anger. Using the word, "I'm awesome, "Remain calm," or "This is not beneficial," again and again will let you in minimizing or decreasing furious thoughts.

- Tension elements can be stretched or massaged. If you are tensing your shoulders, for example, roll them or softly rub down your neck and scalp.

- Count to ten slowly. Concentrate on counting to permit your rational questioning to entice up collectively along with your emotions. Start counting again in case you although experience out of control while you get to ten.

- Try to have interaction in some activity. Anger is fueled via the usage of ruminating about a tough scenario. If you have got were given had a difficult day at art work, as an instance, reviewing the whole lot that went incorrect all middle of the night will go away you locked in a rut. Changing the channel for your mind and focusing on some component else absolutely may be the fine manner to loosen up. It is not continuously effective to tell yourself, "Don't fear about that." Distracting your self with an pastime is the very excellent approach to mentally shift gears. Do something that desires your entire interest and makes it harder for indignant or terrible thoughts to enter your mind.

Deep cleaning the kitchen, gambling with the youngsters, and weeding the garden are only a few examples. Find an hobby to hold yourself occupied so that you do no longer linger on the topics which is probably bothering you. Then your frame and thoughts might be capable of lighten up.

- Try speakme to a friend. Talking out an hassle or expressing your issues to a person who has a calming affect on you may be useful. However, hold in mind that venting can backfire. Complaining about your boss, list all of the motives you dislike someone, or whining about all the plain injustices may additionally moreover additionally upload gasoline to the fireside. It is a commonplace misperception which you want to specific your anger as a way to revel in better.

However, studies shows which you don't need to "get your rage out." When you are livid, smashing devices, as an example, may additionally make you even angrier. As a quit result, it's miles essential to use warning even as using this coping approach. If you're going to talk to a chum approximately some detail, make sure you're working on a solution or lessening your anger in vicinity of sincerely venting. It is unjust to rely on them as a sounding board. Instead, you may discover that speaking about a few aspect aside from the situation that makes you livid is the excellent method to hire this approach.

- Visualize your self being calm. This tip desires you to vicinity your new respiratory techniques into exercising. Close your eyes. Visualize your self calmness after taking more than one deep breaths. Now remember your frame comfortable on the same time as you parent via a strain-inducing situation even as last centered and tranquility. When you create a highbrow demonstration of what it looks as if to be calm, you can flip to it at the same time as you're feeling worried.

- Challenge your questioning. Having irrational mind that do not make experience is a part of being livid or involved. These are typically the "worst-case situation" thoughts. You may additionally moreover additionally get caught inside the "what if" cycle, that may result in you sabotaging essential factors of your existence. Pause and ask yourself the subsequent questions if you have this type of thoughts:

Is this a possibility?

Is this an inexpensive assumption?

What is the worst situation that would display up in fact? Is it some element I can deal with?

- We have all misinterpreted a pal's or associate's commentary, specially on the identical time as we're hungry, fatigued, or careworn. So taking a 2d to undergo in thoughts the genuine cause of a apparently cruel announcement can abruptly calm a scenario. When we get irritated, our mind perceives someone as a danger, and we must shield ourselves, however every so often we interpret subjects incorrect or pay interest things incorrectly.

- It is straightforward to stay in denial and refuse to admit your flaws. Take a minute to assess a mindset that is to your quality pastimes if someone close to you shows it earlier than disregarding it outright and turning into furious. This will become simpler over time when you have an mindset of ongoing improvement. Actively are trying to find grievance; it'll help you make bigger a thick pores and pores and skin and, inside the process, provide you with a present day perspective on matters.

• Take a 2nd. Think approximately all of the belongings you are grateful for. Instead of feeling that the whole thing is wrong, apprehend which you have plenty to be glad about. This may additionally moreover assist you manage your anger.

3.6 Expressing Your Anger in a Healthy Way

The problem is that we aren't taught the manner to explicit ourselves in a healthy way, so we become stuffing our emotions. We are each taught to absolutely avoid our emotions, or we have got were given witnessed a few especially unpleasant expressions of anger, making even considering expression seem terrifying. Whether the anger is directed at your circle of relatives, pals, or coworkers, it wishes to be managed and expressed in a healthful way:

• Start with what we call the "pain caveat" whilst you wish to talk rage or a few special horrible emotion. Make it apparent to others that you are experiencing sturdy emotions and that it is greater hard a very good manner to speak genuinely than everyday. Apologize in advance of time, no longer for your feelings or movements, however for the possibly lack of clarity in how you're going to mention it.

The purpose of the soreness caveat is to de-enhance the situation and prevent the man or woman from becoming protecting. When a person is aware that you are uncomfortable and that the talk is difficult for you, they'll be more likely to listen with empathy to what you have got to mention.

- You is probably able to write what you can't say. Make a listing of the manner you enjoy and the way you need to react. It assist you to loosen up and look at the events that led up on your emotions if you write them down. An anger control pocket ebook is a tool that may be used to help people control their anger. When we are furious, we frequently go through a form of mental "fog" in which our functionality to expect is hampered. Writing in an anger management pocket book assists the thoughts to awareness its mind with the useful resource of allowing it to explicit itself in a considerate and targeted manner. Even virtually "reporting" what made you irritated or the manner it made you sense would possibly help you regain manage of your mind and feelings.

Simultaneously, in reality writing approximately furious emotions and who or what introduced on them is not enough to reap a sense of closure and lengthy-time period manage.

An anger control pocket book need to have shape and emphasis past filling up clean pages with recollections of slights, hurts, and frustrations to make that form of development.

There is no one approach to developing an anger control magazine. However, there are three important factors for optimum performance and very last peace of mind:

Self-Acknowledgment: There isn't always any way to find out a healthy treatment before someone recognizes that there can be a problem. This isn't always to say that your article for your anger control magazine has to test like a confession of a transgression.

Instead, it's far useful to maintain in thoughts topics:

1. A description of your anger in phrases of an emotional reaction (which consist of who or what come to be worried, even as or wherein it happened, and how or why your anger became induced)

2. The situations in that you felt indignant, e.G., who or what have turn out to be worried, whilst or in which it befell, and the manner or why your anger changed into precipitated (use of profanity, physical response, yelling, and lots of others.)

You are validating your self with this acknowledgment, and you're permitting yourself to understand the circumstance and your anger with extra readability with this attitude. Learning and increase emerge via acknowledgment and the following attitude.

Self-Compassion: Many people who are in reality livid cognizance their wrath on themselves, resulting in a devastating and exhausting cycle of resentment and regret.

That is why writing approximately self-compassion in your anger manipulate mag is essential. This isn't to mention that you want to wipe the slate clean or neglect approximately about any lousy outcomes of your anger. Instead, self-compassion is a journaling method that permits you to interrupt the cycle of anger and remorse. You can write for your pocket e-book that everybody receives livid and makes errors and that you are running on regulating your feelings and getting manipulate of your anger. This is a method, and writing such reminders in your mag allow you to to be greater open to receiving and giving compassion and forgiveness. Compassion and forgiveness relieve the giver further to the receiver in their burdens. That is one of the motives there are such plenty of amazing prices on letting skip of grudges and anger. Self-compassion and self-forgiveness supply a lift to our skills to expose compassion and forgiveness to others, easing our emotional burden.

Mindful Action: Journaling approximately thoughtful/conscious motion will help you experience extra cushty and go along with the float forward. This does no longer recommend you want to offer you with a method to repair or mend the very last consequences of your anger, however it is probably a exceptional concept now and again. Creating an entry that displays considerate motion, however, want to include a coping method apart from rage. You can also, as an instance, take a look at your self-compassion and write down the reaction you preference you had alternatively or an idea for a manner to remind your destiny self to halt and breathe earlier than permitting anger to weigh down you.

Overall, this a part of the journaling approach will provide you with a enjoy of closure or decision, allowing you to transport on from the state of affairs and your angry response.

If those sentiments cross again, or in case you locate yourself stuck remembering and reliving specific sports that made you indignant, bypass lower lower returned to this segment of your get entry to and remind your self to preserve shifting in advance for your sports in preference to going backward and interrupting your improvement.

• Improve your communique competencies. Being overly irritated and violent can also need to make it difficult to correctly communicate your emotions and views. People can be preoccupied along side your rage and find out it hard to pay hobby what you are announcing. On the alternative aspect, if you could unique your anger via speakme assertively and respectfully approximately what has made you furious, others are much more likely to understand you.

Being assertive includes sticking up for oneself while additionally respecting the views of others. It may be capable of:

Facilitate conversation

Avert demanding conditions from getting out of manipulate

Boost your conceitedness and connections

It might not seem easy within the starting to learn how to be assertive, however proper here are a few subjects to attempt:

Consider the surrender end stop result you need to accumulate. What irritates you, and what may also you need to exchange? Is it enough to simply usa your complaint?

Be as specific as possible. For instance, you could begin your declaration with, "I am disillusioned with you due to the fact..." Using the term "I feel" avoids assigning blame and makes the opposite individual experience an entire lot tons much less attacked. Respectful and specific conversation is essential. Instead of announcing, "You in no way do any home tasks," say, "I'm disillusioned which you left the desk with out providing to assist with the dishes."

Listen cautiously to the alternative man or woman's response and try and recognize their perspective.

- Be conscious even as the conversation is going off the rails, and try to be conscious whilst this takes vicinity. If you locate yourself turning into enraged, you have to move returned to the communique at a later time.

- Give yourself permission to halt for a time whilst you're upset, although someone is looking forward to a response. You may additionally additionally even tell them which you are deliberately slowing down the situation. Rather than making quick selections, choose to make right ones.

Pauses, deep breaths, and durations of reflected image exercising extra electricity and control than speedy-fireside replies at the same time as you're indignant. If slowing down makes you enjoy a lot less dissatisfied, this is notable, but that is not the point. In an emotionally charged scenario, this is about supplying oneself extra alternatives to choose out from.

- It is straightforward to skip judgment on others; yet, empathy requires effort and time. It is intellectually closed-minded and lazy to make judgments and labels. When you are dissatisfied, take a step again and remember if some factor from your everyday everyday is making you indignant. It can be a few component as simple as adjusting your move from side to side to work or your ordinary duties; a small trade right here and there could make a considerable difference. But, a good way to avoid worry, do now not move too speedy; alternatively, do matters slowly.

- We will be predisposed to mention hurtful topics or terms to someone simply due to the reality we are irritated. To avoid this, take into account rehearsing what you're about to say so you do now not get the identical response the following time.

- When you are disillusioned, it's miles obtrusive that you do no longer have control over your terms. As a stop result, in case you are angry via some element, it's miles awesome to refrain from talking. Most of the time, preserving your mouth close works properly. You will go through a fantastic deal if you pick out to speak over being silent. You want to deal with the alternative man or woman quite and rationally. This method will come up with the 'Freedom to Choose' your solution whilst additionally improving your conceitedness in the long run. When you chorus from passing judgment on others, you are much less willing to skip judgment on your self.

- Throwing a few difficulty can help reduce stress and be beneficial inside the quick time period. Do you've got got a outdoor? If you have were given enough room, get to be had with a ball or some rocks to throw. Alternatively, destroy some thing you preferred to get rid of, which encompass a mug or an vintage piece of garbage. If that isn't always an alternative, get inventive and hurl a few factor clean (together with a roll of relaxation room paper or balled-up socks) inside the route of a clean wall or into the woods.

- Consider your self a chess participant. Consider how the other character will reply and the way the situation will appearance moves from now earlier than selecting a route of motion. Continue to your modern-day-day-day adventure if everything seems to be in order. Consider an exchange behavior, photograph how they'll reply, and examine this state of affairs if it appears to be horrible.

- When you feel enraged, yelling into your pillow may be immensely cathartic and help you get out of your rage. If you are at artwork and feature a few minutes to spare, your car is likewise a probable desire.

- Rather than specializing in what made you irritated, awareness on resolving the modern-day hassle. Is your little one's strewn-about room using you insane? Close the door in the once more of you. Is your boyfriend constantly late for dinner? Plan your food for a bit later in the night — or comply with dine on my own a couple of instances in step with week. Remind your self that anger is not going to treatment some thing and can even make subjects worse. If you accept as true with you can change your present day function, the first step is to just accept responsibility to your contemporary-day-day situation. People who are proactive accumulate an answer-oriented mind-set through the years and as a end result spend much much less time in the first diploma of rage.

- Do not harbor a grudge in competition to anyone. Forgiveness is a really powerful weapon. Allowing anger and one of a kind lousy feelings to overpower satisfied feelings may bring about you being swept up by means of your very very very own bitterness or revel in of unfairness. However, if you could forgive a person who has indignant you, you'll be capable of have a take a look at from the occasion at the same time as additionally strengthening your friendship.

These are the six essential steps in an effort to will let you manipulate your anger and lead a calm, peaceful existence.

Chapter 8: Managing a Stressed Brain

Effective stress control permit you to harm the shackles that stress has to your life, enabling you to be healthier, happier, and extra efficient. What we want is a balanced life amongst relationships, paintings, fun, and rest, and to increase the electricity to preserve going while topics get hard. Stress control has many strategies of which a few may match for you and some may not. That is why it's miles essential to try numerous matters and discern out what works for you.

Let's debunk some myths approximately pressure in advance than we waft ahead.

- Stress is all spherical you, and there may be no longer some factor you can do about it.

True, stress is all spherical us, however you could manage your life such that it does now not consume you. Setting priorities and fixing number one problems first in advance than tackling greater complex disturbing conditions is a extraordinary technique. When we are careworn, it is hard to prioritize because all problems seem like further distressing.

- Only the maximum intense pressure signs and signs want to be addressed.

Minor symptoms and symptoms and symptoms, which encompass headaches or belly acid, are early caution symptoms and signs that your life is out of manipulate and must not be overlooked. Do now not wait till a immoderate strain symptom, e.G., a coronary heart attack, to get assist; it may already be too past due. Making life-style changes, at the side of getting greater workout or consuming a greater wholesome diet plan will save you time, cash and enhance your fitness. Furthermore, if signs and symptoms are not controlled, stress can rapid improvement from acute to persistent.

- Stress may be used as a motivator.

Although some humans are inspired through pressure, the benefits of motivation do not exceed the overall negative impact on fitness. Chinese community health experts were asked about their paintings strain and motivation in connection to procedure pride in a 2014 poll . This take a look at placed that paintings-associated strain had a bad relationship with project pleasure using separate requirements.

Short-time period stress, especially acute pressure, can be motivating for a few people. Acute strain improves an individual's alertness and allows them whole responsibilities along side mission key closing dates. Acute stress can also assist humans in acting at their excellent and wondering imaginatively approximately how to triumph over problems. Stress is justified as a motivator in a few situations.

Chronic pressure, however, which has extended-time period poor results, is less of a motivator and extra of a burden. The lengthy-time period dangers of persistent pressure on someone's physical, mental, and emotional nicely-being outweighs the advantages of acute strain.

- If there aren't any signs and symptoms and symptoms and symptoms or symptoms and symptoms, there may be no pressure.

Just because of the reality someone does now not display off strain-associated symptoms or signs and signs and symptoms does not recommend that they will be now not compelled. Stress can fast appear itself in a few humans via behavioral adjustments or after annoying occurrences. However, it could be fantastically tough to tell if a few are forced, based totally completely mostly on their conduct. Such human beings may additionally additionally appear regular and cover their tension correctly, but they will be clearly suffering with emotionally. Stress is normally manifested in methods: cognitively and emotionally.

The following pressure management techniques allow you to to your pressure-unfastened adventure:

4.1 Identifying Source of Stress

Exploring the reasons within the again of your burdened life is the primary step in strain management. However, figuring them out might not be straightforward. While massive stresses like moving, changing jobs, or going thru a divorce are clean to phrase, spotting the origins of persistent strain may be very tough. It is simple to misconceive the detail that your private emotions, mind, and behaviors have in your pressure tiers. You can be continuously involved approximately paintings cut-off dates, however it is possible that the strain is as a result of your procrastination in choice to the real challenge obligations.

Examine your behaviors, mind-set, and excuses to determine your actual belongings of stress:

• Do you watched of pressure as part of your system or home lifestyles ("Things are continually a piece frantic spherical right right right here") or as a man or woman trait ("I in reality have pretty some demanding power that is all")?

- Do you rationalize your strain as temporary ("I without a doubt have a million matters on my plate proper now"), regardless of the fact which you can't recall the very last time you took a destroy?

- Do you accept as true with you studied your stress is delivered on due to different humans or out of doors activities, or do you believe you studied it's far virtually unexceptional and ordinary?

Your stress will stay out of your control till you're taking shipping of obligation on your detail in inflicting or perpetuating it.

Keeping a Stress Journal Will Help You Understand Your Problem

Keeping a pocket book or diary is extra than only a device to file your thoughts and evaluations. Journaling is an effective strain comfort exercise, regular with cutting-edge research, and those who write in a diary or different pocket book get preserve of every physical and emotional blessings, probable extending their lives.

When as compared to a control institution, psychotherapy patients who have been knowledgeable to precise their feelings through expressive writing had decrease anxiety and depression symptoms and symptoms and made more improvement in psychotherapy, steady with a contemporary have a have a look at posted in Psychotherapy Research.

Journaling can also assist you in decreasing the quantity of worry you revel in. Another have a look at published within the mag Behavior Modification determined that expressive writing became associated with terrific reductions in signs and symptoms and signs of generalized tension infection, collectively with despair and fear.

How to do it?

Some human beings find out putting pen to paper to be healing, at the equal time as others choose typing their thoughts into a computer. There are even Web internet internet web sites that allow human beings to mag privately online, collectively with LiveJournal and Penzu.

Take a while for your self in a peaceful, comfortable region in which you may now not be disturbed. Simply start writing and date your magazine get entry to. When it includes journaling, there aren't any hard and speedy recommendations. You can write some factor which you need. You ought to make your diary get entry to as long or as brief as you pick out. Because nobody but you may have a look at your journal, don't worry approximately language or punctuation; definitely report your mind as they stand up to you. It is hard to understand in which to start even as writing a diary access, however writing approximately your everyday sports is a incredible method to get your thoughts flowing.

Remember that writing about your thoughts, hopes, issues, frustrations, and any other feelings you are experiencing to your pocket book can be a awesome pressure reliever, so try and write approximately them.

A pressure mag let you in figuring out your regular stressors and the way you address them. Keep a pocket e book or use a pressure tracker to your phone to preserve song of your strain degrees. You may be able to see patterns and not unusual triggers in case you keep a every day log. Try to comprise the subsequent subjects that will help you make experience of your pressure:

- What end up the deliver of your pressure? (Guess in case you are not certain)

- How you physically and emotionally felt?

- How you reacted to the situation?

- What you probably did to sense higher?

four.2 Being Aware of Stress Signs

Although it is able to appear self-apparent that you could tell on the identical time as you are harassed, loads folks spend a lot time frazzled that we have forgotten what it is like when our concerned structures are in stability: even as we are calm but alert and centered. If this describes you, listening to your body will let you stumble on at the same time as you're confused. Your eyes may also revel in heavy, and you could lay your head to your hand whilst you are fatigued. When you're glad, it is straightforward to chortle. When you are careworn, your frame can even will let you comprehend. Make it a exercising to pay heed to your frame's signs.

- Examine your frame: Do you have got stiff or aching muscle mass? Do you have got a first rate, cramped, or painful stomach? Do you have clenched hands or a clenched jaw?

- Pay interest on your breathing: Is it difficult that lets in you to take a deep breath? One hand ought to be on your belly, while the other should be on your chest. With each breath, study how your fingers rise and fall. Keep tune of even as you completely breathe and on the same time as you "neglect" to respire.

4. Three Finding Response for a Quick Stress Relief

Internally, the "combat-or-flight" pressure reaction reasons your blood stress to growth, your coronary heart to beat faster, and your muscle agencies to constrict. Your immune device is depleted due to your frame's hard artwork. People, on the other hand, react to pressure in one in each of a kind techniques at the out of doors.

The greatest approach to alleviate strain rapidly is to apprehend your pressure response:

• If you're vulnerable to being livid, overly emotional, agitated, or demanding whilst you are pressured, you may advantage from strain-relieving sports activities activities that may calm you down.

- If you are vulnerable to being unhappy, withdrawn, or spaced out whilst you are pressured, you can advantage from pressure-relieving sports activities which might be appealing and lively.

Do you recognize approximately the "frozen" or the immobilization response?

A history of trauma is frequently associated with the immobilization stress response. When confronted with stressful conditions, you may experience virtually trapped and powerless to act. Your purpose is to reboot your apprehensive gadget and reactivate the frame's herbal "fight-or-flight" stress reaction in order to break unfastened from your "frozen" function. Walking, swimming, sprinting, mountain climbing or tai chi are all examples of bodily sports that make use of each your arms and legs. Instead of focusing for your thoughts, cope with your frame and the feelings you enjoy for your limbs as you skip. This mindfulness aspect also can help your concerned device is becoming "unstuck" and moving beforehand.

Use Your Senses

You must first decide which sensory studies are maximum beneficial to you. This can also necessitate a few trial and errors. Keep music of the manner rapid your stress stages lower as you use exclusive senses. Also, be as accurate as feasible. What is the proper sound or motion that has the most impact on you?

Explore diverse sensory critiques so that you will generally have a stress-relieving tool no matter in which you're. The following samples are alleged to function an area to start. Allow your mind to run wild as you offer you with new things to test. You will recognise if you have determined the right sensory technique. • Manage your mind. Your anger is fueled by way of angry thoughts. "I can't stand it," you would possibly suppose. "This website online traffic delay goes to break the whole thing," you can expect to yourself. Reframe your mind at the same time as you find yourself thinking about subjects that make you indignant. Instead, take into account the data and provide a few component like, "Every day, heaps and loads of motors are on the street." There might be traffic jams on occasion." Staying calmer can be as easy as focusing on the records with out throwing in terrible prophecies or twisted exaggerations. You might also provide you with a mantra that you could repeat to drown out the thoughts which can be fueling your anger. Using the phrase, "I'm first-class, "Remain calm," or "This isn't useful," repeatedly let you in minimizing or decreasing furious thoughts.

• Tension factors may be stretched or massaged. If you are tensing your shoulders, for instance, roll them or softly massage your neck and scalp.

• Count to 10 slowly. Concentrate on counting to permit your rational wondering to trap up collectively along side your feelings. Start counting another time in case you nevertheless enjoy out of manipulate at the same time as you get to 10.

•	Try to engage in a few interest. Anger is fueled through ruminating approximately a tough state of affairs. If you've got had a difficult day at art work, for instance, reviewing the entirety that went incorrect all midnight will leave you locked in a rut. Changing the channel in your thoughts and focusing on something else in reality can be the first-rate way to loosen up. It isn't always commonly effective to tell your self, "Don't worry about that." Distracting your self with an hobby is the perfect approach to mentally shift gears. Do a few thing that dreams your entire interest and makes it more difficult for angry or negative thoughts to enter your mind.

Deep cleansing the kitchen, playing with the children, and weeding the garden are only a few examples. Find an hobby to keep your self occupied so you do not linger at the matters which are bothering you. Then your body and mind can be able to loosen up.

- Try talking to a chum. Talking out an trouble or expressing your worries to someone who has a relaxing have an effect on on you'll be useful. However, preserve in mind that venting can backfire. Complaining approximately your boss, list all the reasons you dislike someone, or whining approximately all the obvious injustices may additionally moreover add gas to the hearth. It is a common misperception that you want to particular your anger if you need to revel in higher.

However, research indicates which you do no longer need to "get your rage out." When you are furious, smashing gadgets, for example, may moreover make you even angrier. As a end end end result, it's far critical to apply caution on the equal time as using this coping method. If you're going to talk to a friend approximately something, ensure you're going for walks on a solution or lessening your anger in desire to truly venting. It is unjust to depend upon them as a sounding board. Instead, you will likely discover that speakme about some issue other than the state of affairs that makes you furious is the satisfactory technique to hire this technique.

• Visualize yourself being calm. This tip wishes you to location your new respiration techniques into exercise. Close your eyes. Visualize yourself calmness after taking multiple deep breaths. Now do not forget your body snug at the same time as you figure through a stress-inducing situation on the equal time as remaining targeted and calmness. When you create a highbrow demonstration of what it looks like to be calm, you may turn to it at the same time as you feel concerned.

• Challenge your questioning. Having irrational mind that don't make sense is part of being furious or concerned. These are commonly the "worst-case state of affairs" thoughts. You might also get stuck inside the "what if" cycle, that might bring about you sabotaging essential factors of your existence. Pause and ask yourself the following questions when you have this form of mind:

Is this a opportunity?

Is this an cheap assumption?

What is the worst state of affairs that could display up in truth? Is it some factor I can cope with?

- We have all misinterpreted a chum's or partner's observation, in particular while we're hungry, fatigued, or burdened. So taking a 2d to undergo in mind the real cause of a apparently merciless remark can rapidly calm a scenario. When we get angry, our thoughts perceives someone as a chance, and we should protect ourselves, however sometimes we interpret things incorrect or hear matters incorrectly.

- It is straightforward to live in denial and refuse to confess your flaws. Take a minute to evaluate a attitude this is in your top notch pastimes if someone near you shows it earlier than disregarding it outright and turning into furious. This will become much much less complicated over time when you have an mindset of ongoing development. Actively are trying to find complaint; it's going to help you boom a thick skin and, in the method, offer you with a modern-day mind-set on topics.

• Take a 2nd. Think about all of the things you are thankful for. Instead of feeling that the entirety is incorrect, apprehend that you have masses to be glad approximately. This also can help you manage your anger.

three.6 Expressing Your Anger in a Healthy Way

The problem is that we aren't taught the manner to explicit ourselves in a wholesome way, so we turn out to be stuffing our emotions. We are both taught to virtually avoid our emotions, or we've got witnessed some highly unpleasant expressions of anger, making even thinking about expression seem terrifying. Whether the anger is directed at your circle of relatives, pals, or coworkers, it desires to be controlled and expressed in a wholesome manner:

- Start with what we call the "pain caveat" even as you choice to talk rage or a few other horrible emotion. Make it obvious to others that you are experiencing robust emotions and that it is extra hard to be able to talk in reality than everyday. Apologize in advance of time, no longer to your emotions or movements, but for the in all likelihood loss of readability in how you're going to mention it.

The motive of the pain caveat is to de-pork up the state of affairs and save you the individual from becoming defensive. When a person is conscious that you are uncomfortable and that the talk is difficult for you, they'll be much more likely to pay attention with empathy to what you have to say.

- You might be capable of write what you cannot say. Make a list of the manner you sense and how you need to react. It permit you to lighten up and study the occasions that led up in your emotions in case you write them down. An anger control pocket e book is a device that may be used to assist humans control their anger. When we are livid, we regularly undergo a shape of intellectual "fog" wherein our capability to think is hampered. Writing in an anger manage pocket e-book assists the mind to hobby its mind thru allowing it to specific itself in a thoughtful and centered way. Even absolutely "reporting" what made you indignant or the way it made you sense may moreover help you regain manipulate of your mind and feelings.

Simultaneously, actually writing approximately livid feelings and who or what triggered them isn't sufficient to reap a experience of closure and prolonged-time period manage.

An anger manage pocket e-book want to have shape and emphasis past filling up easy pages with stories of slights, hurts, and frustrations to make that shape of improvement.

There isn't anybody technique to growing an anger manage mag. However, there are three critical factors for optimum common performance and ultimate peace of mind:

Self-Acknowledgment: There isn't any manner to find out a healthy treatment before someone acknowledges that there can be a problem. This is not to say that your article on your anger control mag has to take a look at like a confession of a transgression.

Instead, it's miles useful to consider topics:

1.   A description of your anger in phrases of an emotional response (which includes who or what changed into worried, even as or wherein it befell, and the way or why your anger have become introduced on)

2.   The events in which you felt angry, e.G., who or what end up involved, while or in which it befell, and the way or why your anger became brought on (use of profanity, bodily response, yelling, and masses of others.)

You are validating your self with this acknowledgment, and you're allowing yourself to recognize the circumstance and your anger with greater readability with this attitude. Learning and increase emerge via acknowledgment and the following attitude.

Self-Compassion: Many folks that are really livid focus their wrath on themselves, ensuing in a devastating and exhausting cycle of resentment and remorse.

That is why writing about self-compassion in your anger manage mag is critical. This isn't always to mention which you need to wipe the slate easy or neglect approximately any horrible outcomes of your anger. Instead, self-compassion is a journaling approach that allows you to interrupt the cycle of anger and regret. You can write for your pocket book that everybody gets livid and makes mistakes and that you are strolling on regulating your emotions and getting manage of your anger. This is a device, and writing such reminders to your magazine allow you to to be greater open to receiving and giving compassion and forgiveness. Compassion and forgiveness relieve the giver in addition to the receiver of their burdens. That is one of the reasons there are so many remarkable costs on letting skip of grudges and anger. Self-compassion and self-forgiveness assist our capabilities to show compassion and forgiveness to others, easing our emotional burden.

Mindful Action: Journaling about thoughtful/conscious movement will assist you revel in greater at ease and circulate beforehand. This does now not suggest you need to provide you with a method to restore or mend the outcome of your anger, but it is probably a very good idea from time to time. Creating an access that indicates thoughtful action, instead, need to contain a coping approach aside from rage. You may additionally, for instance, check yourself-compassion and write down the response you want you had as an possibility or an concept for the manner to remind your future self to halt and breathe in advance than permitting anger to weigh down you.

Chapter 9: Avert demanding situations from getting out of manipulate

Boost your arrogance and connections

It might not seem easy before the entirety to learn how to be assertive, but right right here are some subjects to attempt:

Consider the save you cease result you want to acquire. What irritates you, and what may you want to trade? Is it enough to truly country your complaint?

Be as unique as viable. For example, you can start your statement with, "I am disappointed with you due to the truth..." Using the time period "I sense" avoids assigning blame and makes the opposite person feel lots much less attacked. Respectful and particular conversation is critical. Instead of saying, "You in no manner do any housekeeping," say, "I'm dissatisfied which you left the desk with out imparting to assist with the dishes."

Listen cautiously to the alternative man or woman's response and try and understand their factor of view.

- Be aware at the identical time because the communication goes off the rails, and try and word when this takes place. If you discover your self becoming enraged, you want to go back to the communique at a later time.

- Give your self permission to halt for a time at the same time as you're disillusioned, even though a person is calling in advance to a reaction. You can also even inform them which you are intentionally slowing down the scenario. Rather than making short picks, pick out out to make accurate ones. Pauses, deep breaths, and intervals of mirrored photo exercising more power and manage than fast-fireplace replies at the same time as you are indignant. If slowing down makes you enjoy much less disenchanted, that is splendid, but that is not the point. In an emotionally charged scenario, that is approximately offering oneself greater options to choose out from.

- It is easy to pass judgment on others; but, empathy calls for time and effort. It is intellectually closed-minded and lazy to make judgments and labels. When you're disenchanted, take a step again and preserve in thoughts if a few element out of your regular recurring is making you indignant. It can be something as smooth as adjusting your go to and fro to artwork or your ordinary responsibilities; a small alternate right right right here and there should make a sizeable difference. But, in case you need to keep away from worry, do not bypass too fast; as an alternative, do subjects slowly.

- We have a propensity to mention hurtful subjects or phrases to a person clearly because of the truth we are angry. To avoid this, do not forget rehearsing what you are about to say so that you do not get the identical reaction the following time.

- When you're disenchanted, it is evident which you do not have control over your words. As a cease end result, if you are irritated thru way of something, it's far tremendous to chorus from speaking. Most of the time, keeping your mouth close works properly. You will go through a awesome deal in case you choose to talk over being silent. You want to treat the opposite individual quite and rationally. This technique will provide you with the 'Freedom to Choose' your solution on the equal time as moreover improving your self-esteem ultimately. When you chorus from passing judgment on others, you're plenty a lot less willing to skip judgment on your self.

- Throwing a few aspect can assist reduce stress and be useful within the short time period. Do you have a outdoor? If you have got were given sufficient room, get available with a ball or some rocks to throw. Alternatively, smash something you desired to cast off, along side a mug or an vintage piece of rubbish. If that isn't always an alternative, get resourceful and hurl some component mild (which encompass a roll of rest room paper or balled-up socks) towards a easy wall or into the woods.

- Consider your self a chess player. Consider how the opposite person will reply and the manner the scenario will appearance moves from now before deciding on a route of motion. Continue in your modern-day journey if the whole thing appears to be so as. Consider an exchange behavior, image how they'll respond, and analyze this state of affairs if it appears to be lousy.

- When you are feeling enraged, yelling into your pillow can be immensely cathartic and help you get out of your rage. If you are at paintings and feature a couple of minutes to spare, your automobile is likewise a feasible choice.

- Rather than that specialize in what made you angry, popularity on resolving the modern-day-day trouble. Is your toddler's strewn-approximately room driving you insane? Close the door inside the once more of you. Is your boyfriend usually past due for dinner? Plan your food for a piece later within the nighttime — or observe dine on my own a couple of times in line with week. Remind yourself that anger isn't always going to clear up anything and can even make matters worse. If you accept as true with you could trade your present function, step one is to accept obligation on your contemporary condition. People who are proactive gather an answer-oriented mindset through the years and as a quit end result spend tons much less time in the first degree of rage.

- Do now not harbor a grudge in the direction of each person. Forgiveness is a very powerful weapon. Allowing anger and other horrible feelings to overpower glad feelings may purpose you being swept up with the aid of the use of your very very very own bitterness or enjoy of unfairness. However, if you may forgive someone who has irritated you, you may be capable to investigate from the occasion on the identical time as moreover strengthening your friendship.

These are the six important steps that permit you to manipulate your anger and lead a cushty, non violent existence.

Managing a Stressed Brain

Effective pressure control allow you to destroy the shackles that strain has on your existence, permitting you to be extra wholesome, happier, and greater green. What we need is a balanced existence among relationships, art work, fun, and rest, and to growth the strength to preserve going while subjects get difficult. Stress manipulate has many strategies of which a few may work for you and a few might not. That is why it is essential to strive different things and parent out what works for you.

Let's debunk some myths approximately pressure before we flow into beforehand.

•	Stress is all round you, and there is not anything you may do approximately it.

True, strain is all spherical us, however you can manage your life such that it does now not consume you. Setting priorities and solving easy troubles first earlier than tackling extra complicated annoying situations is a notable approach. When we're stressed, it's miles difficult to prioritize because all concerns seem like in addition distressing.

- Only the maximum important pressure signs and symptoms and signs and signs and symptoms need to be addressed.

Minor symptoms, such as headaches or stomach acid, are early warning signs that your lifestyles is out of control and need to no longer be ignored. Do not wait until a crucial strain symptom, e.G., a coronary coronary coronary heart attack, to get assist; it can already be too past due. Making way of life adjustments, which include getting greater exercising or consuming a more fit eating regimen will save you time, cash and enhance your health. Furthermore, if signs are not controlled, stress can quick development from acute to chronic.

- Stress can be used as a motivator.

Although some people are inspired by way of the usage of stress, the benefits of motivation do no longer exceed the general negative impact on health. Chinese network fitness professionals had been requested approximately their artwork strain and motivation in connection to technique pride in a 2014 ballot . This test decided that paintings-related strain had a terrible relationship with manner pride the usage of separate requirements.

Short-term strain, particularly acute stress, may be motivating for some people. Acute stress improves an man or woman's alertness and permits them whole obligations which incorporates attaining key time limits. Acute strain also can moreover assist people in acting at their nice and thinking imaginatively approximately how to conquer issues. Stress is justified as a motivator in a few conditions.

Chronic strain, however, which has prolonged-term terrible outcomes, is a incredible deal less of a motivator and similarly of a burden. The long-term dangers of continual pressure on a person's bodily, intellectual, and emotional well-being outweighs the advantages of acute strain.

- If there are no signs and symptoms and signs and symptoms or signs and symptoms, there can be no stress.

Just due to the fact a person does not show off pressure-related symptoms and symptoms or symptoms does not propose that they're not confused. Stress can brief seem itself in a few people via behavioral modifications or after annoying occurrences. However, it is able to be extensively tough to inform if some are harassed, primarily based on their conduct. Such human beings may additionally appear normal and disguise their anxiety effectively, but they may be truly struggling with emotionally. Stress is usually manifested in techniques: cognitively and emotionally.

The following strain manipulate techniques allow you to on your strain-free journey:

four.1 Identifying Source of Stress

Exploring the motives at the back of your pressured existence is the number one step in strain control. However, figuring them out might not be sincere. While large stresses like transferring, changing jobs, or going thru a divorce are easy to observe, recognizing the origins of chronic stress can be very hard. It is easy to misunderstand the detail that your very own feelings, thoughts, and behaviors should your stress levels. You may be usually concerned approximately art work closing dates, but it is viable that the pressure is attributable to your procrastination instead of the real project obligations.

www.ingramcontent.com/pod-product-compliance
Lightning Source LLC
Chambersburg PA
CBHW071124130526
44590CB00056B/1903